THE BEST
ANATOMY
COLORING BOOK

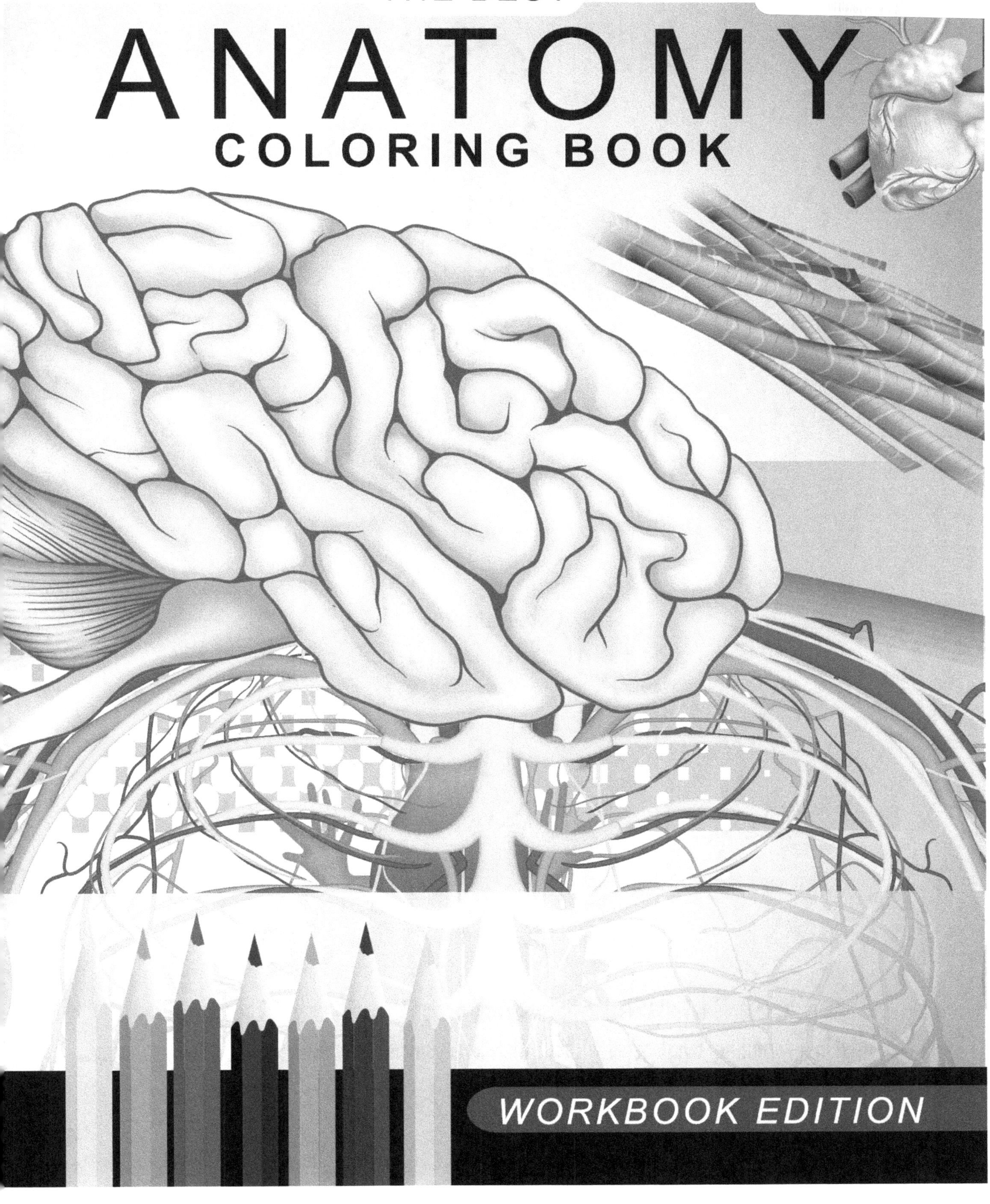

WORKBOOK EDITION

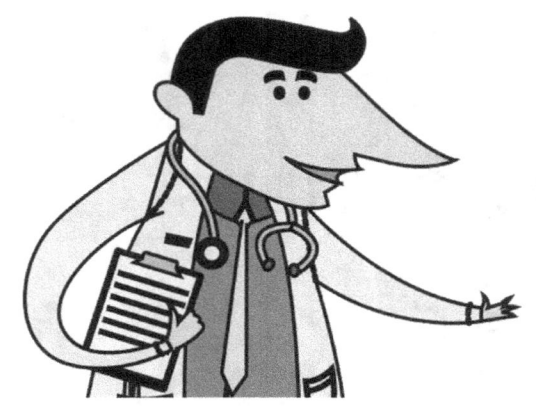

SMART DOCTOR

Copyright 2017
Printed in The U.S.A.

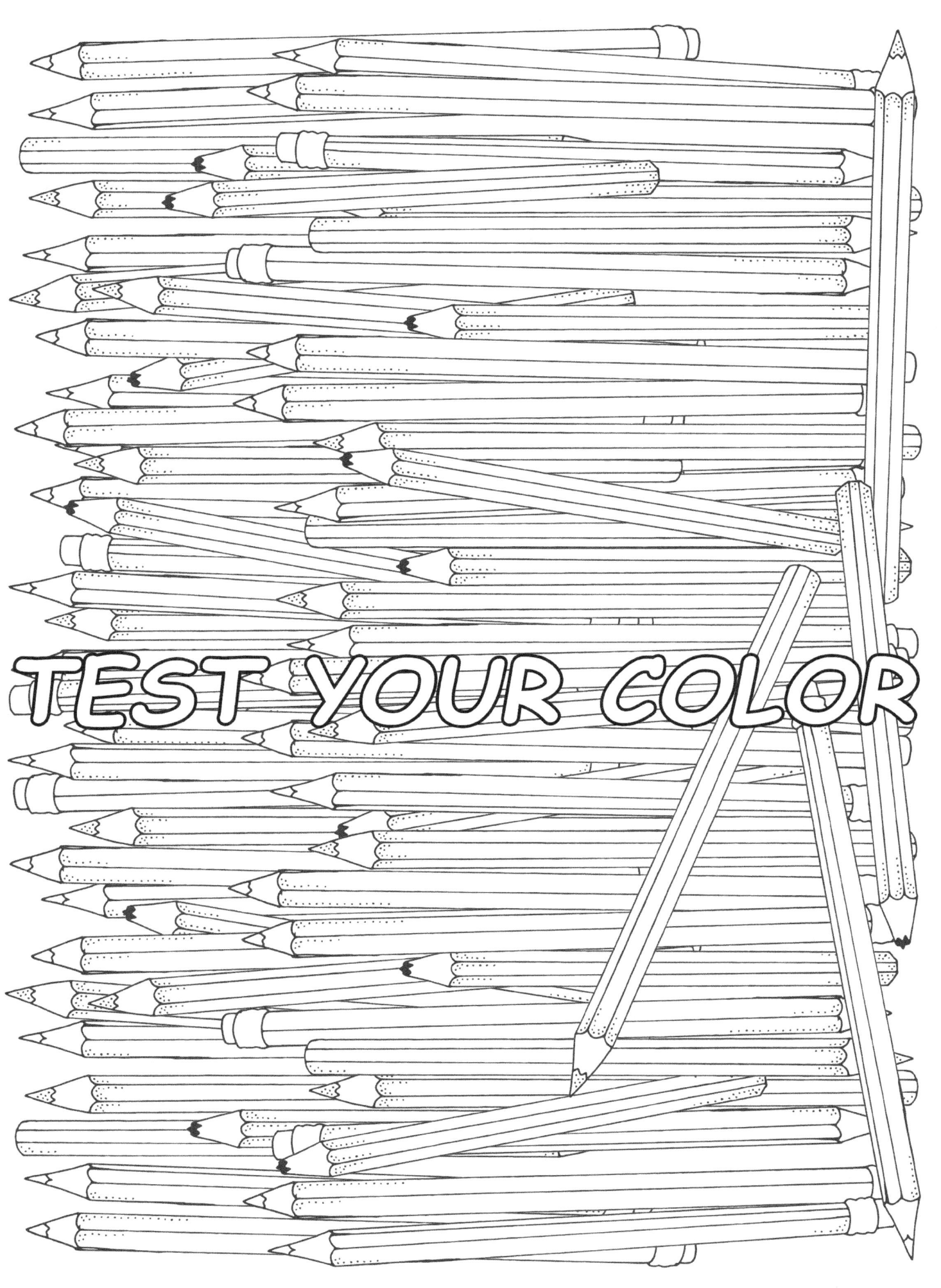

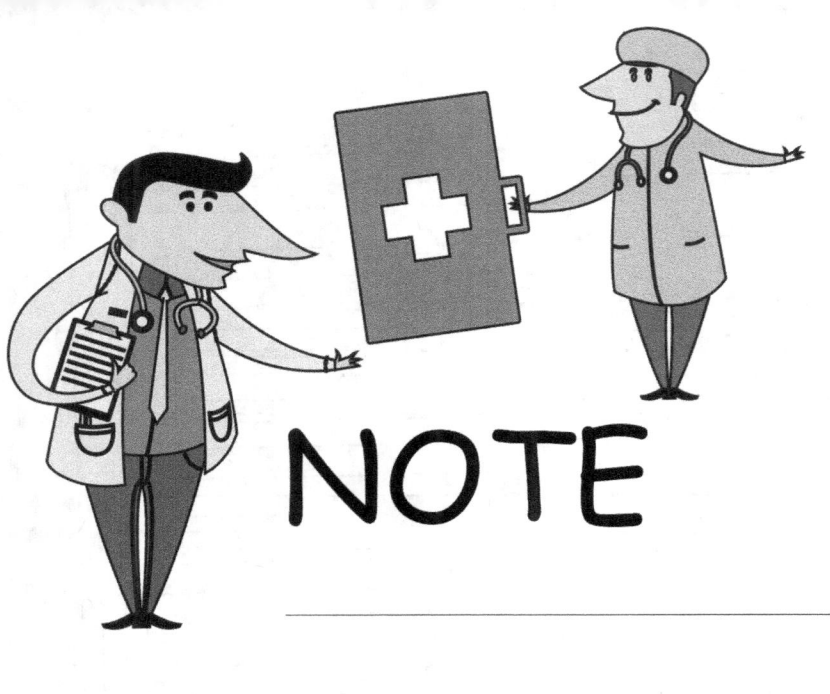

NOTE

SKULL

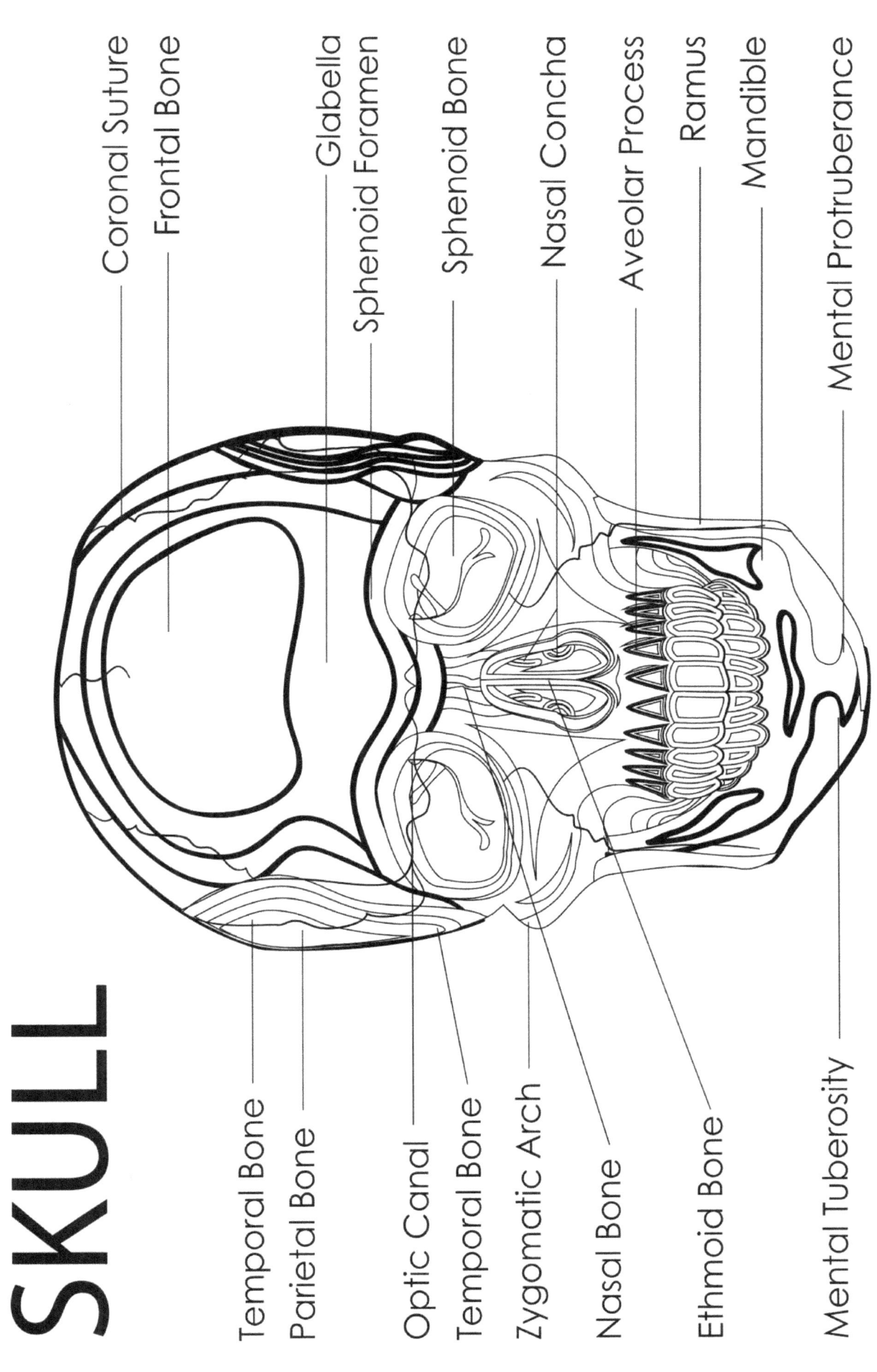

Coronal Suture

Frontal Bone

Glabella

Sphenoid Foramen

Sphenoid Bone

Nasal Concha

Aveolar Process

Ramus

Mandible

Mental Protruberance

Temporal Bone

Parietal Bone

Optic Canal

Temporal Bone

Zygomatic Arch

Nasal Bone

Ethmoid Bone

Mental Tuberosity

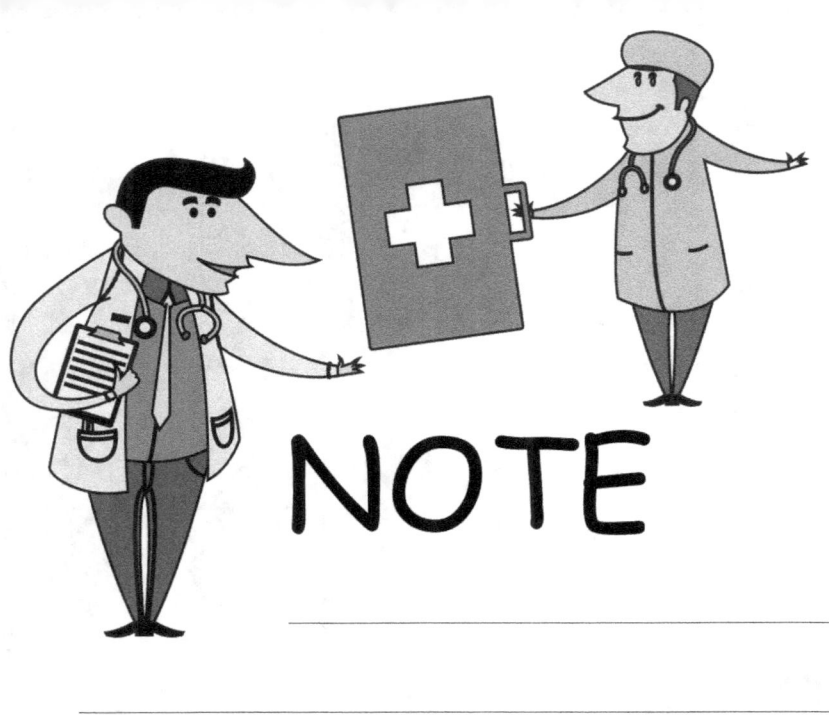

NOTE

BRAIN

Central Sulcus

Parietal Lobe

Lateral Ventricles

Corpus Callosum

Thalamus

Arbor Vitae

Fourth Ventricle

Cerebellum

Cerebellar Cortex

Cerebral Cortex

Frontal Lobe

Hypothalamus

Temporal Lobe

Pituitary Gland

Pons

Medulla

Spinal Cord

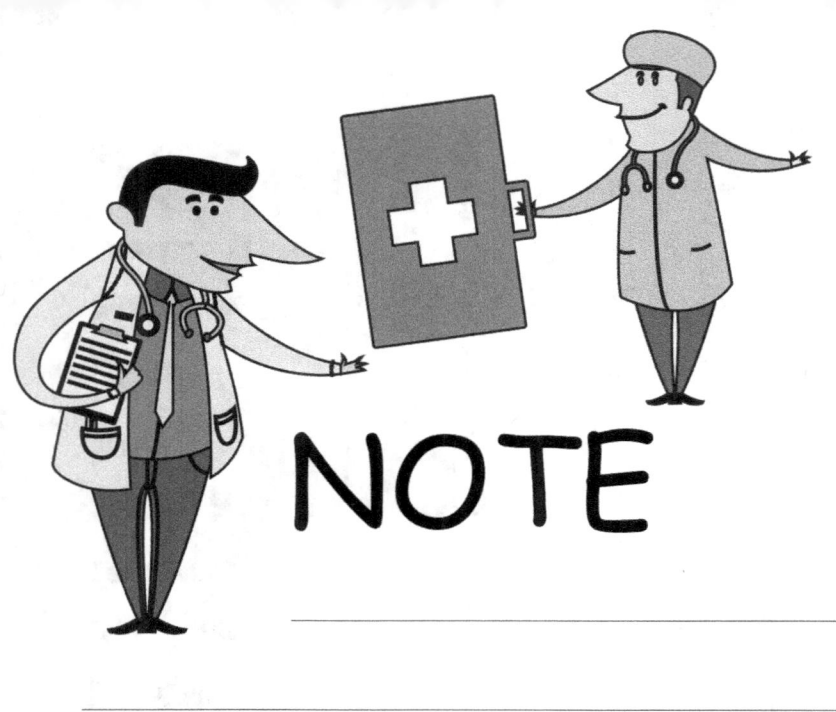

NOTE

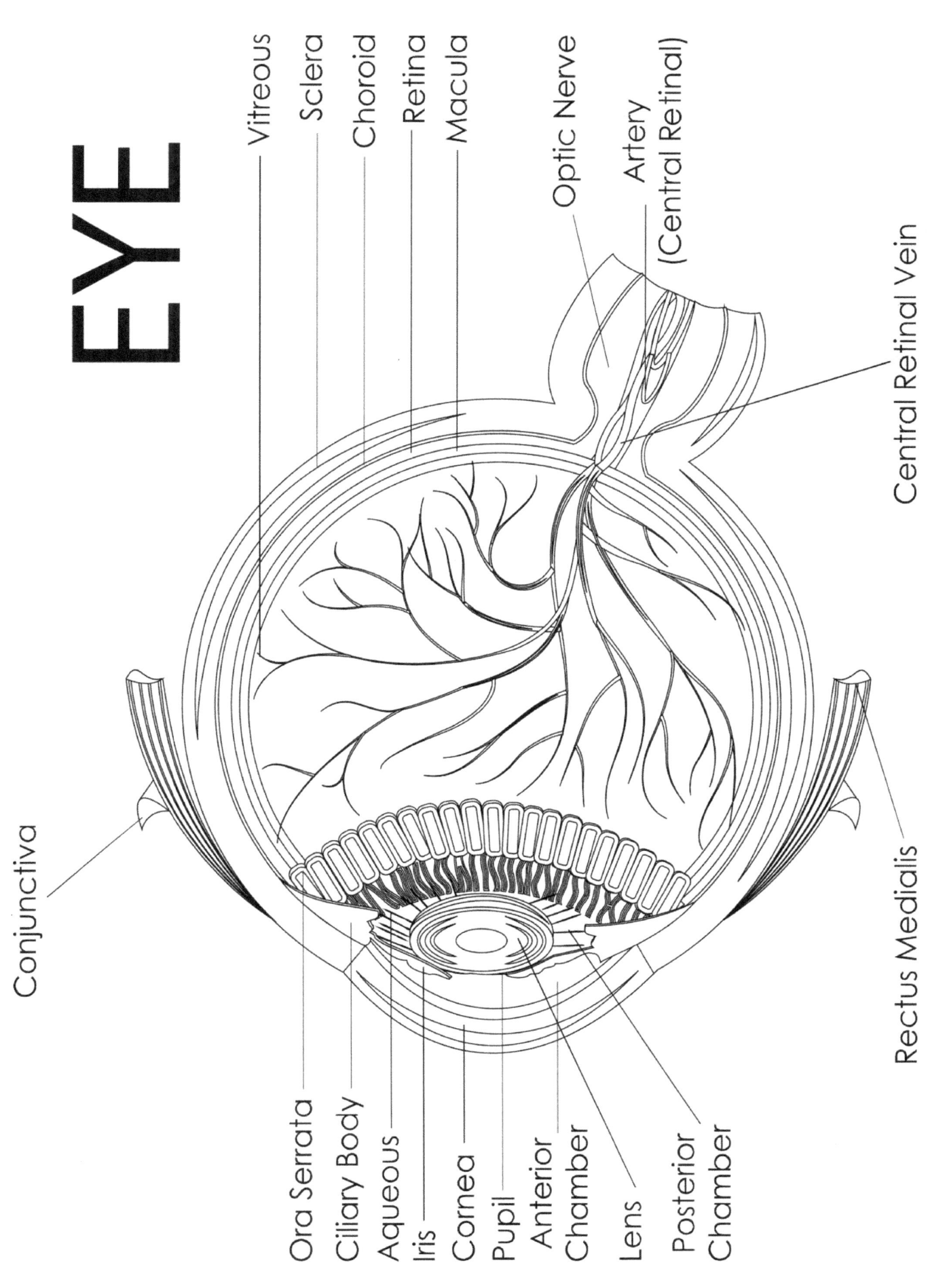

EYE

Vitreous
Sclera
Choroid
Retina
Macula

Optic Nerve

Artery
(Central Retinal)

Central Retinal Vein

Conjunctiva

Ora Serrata
Ciliary Body
Aqueous
Iris
Cornea
Pupil
Anterior
Chamber
Lens
Posterior
Chamber

Rectus Medialis

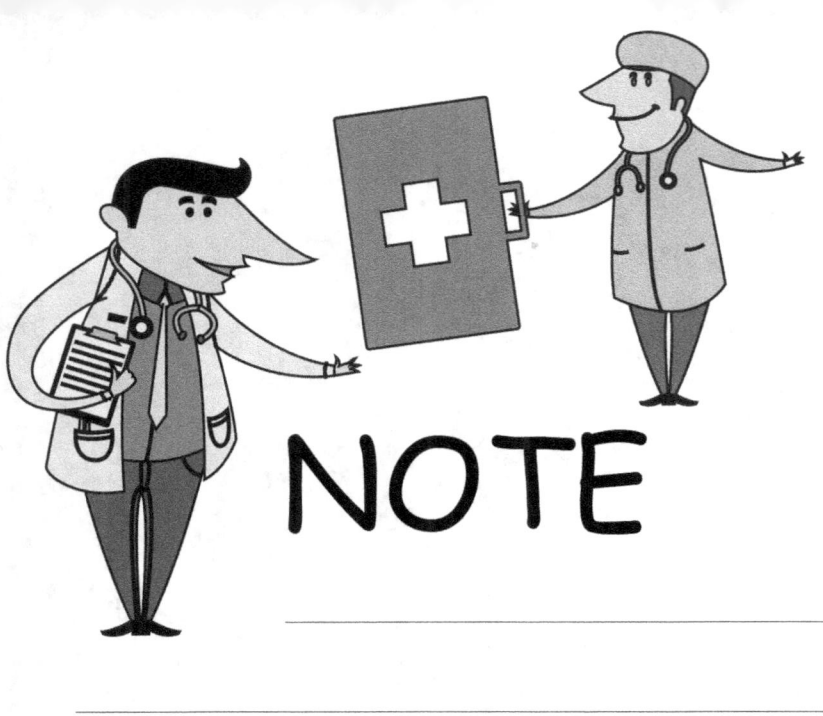

NOTE

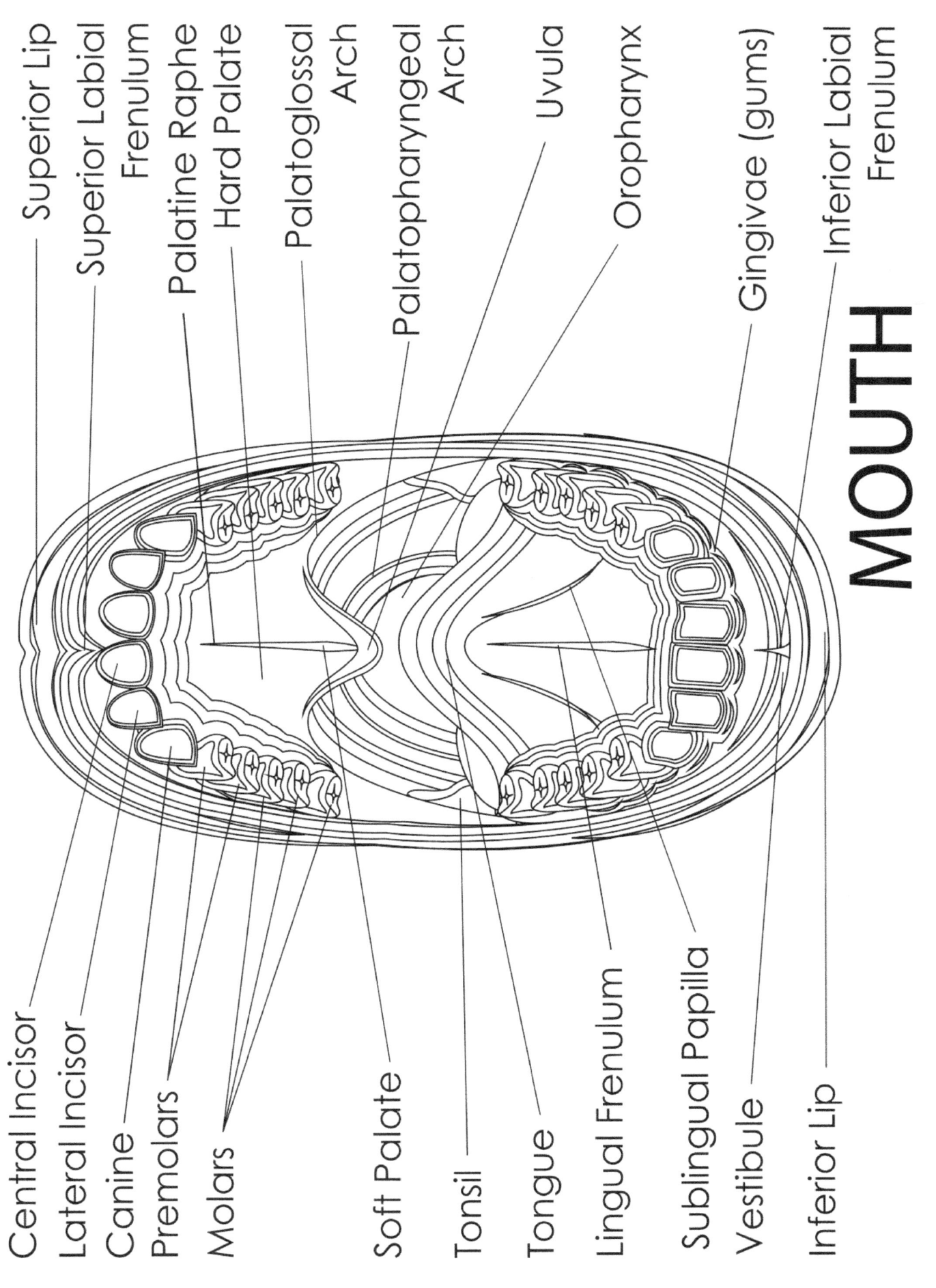

Central Incisor

Lateral Incisor

Canine

Premolars

Molars

Soft Palate

Tonsil

Tongue

Lingual Frenulum

Sublingual Papilla

Vestibule

Inferior Lip

Superior Lip

Superior Labial Frenulum

Palatine Raphe

Hard Palate

Palatoglossal Arch

Palatopharyngeal Arch

Uvula

Oropharynx

Gingivae (gums)

Inferior Labial Frenulum

MOUTH

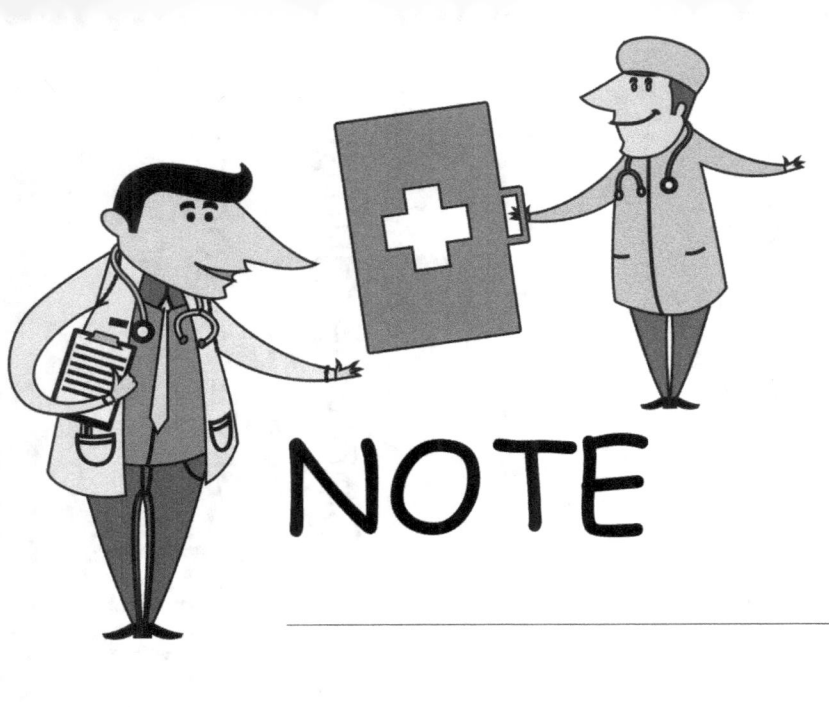

NOTE

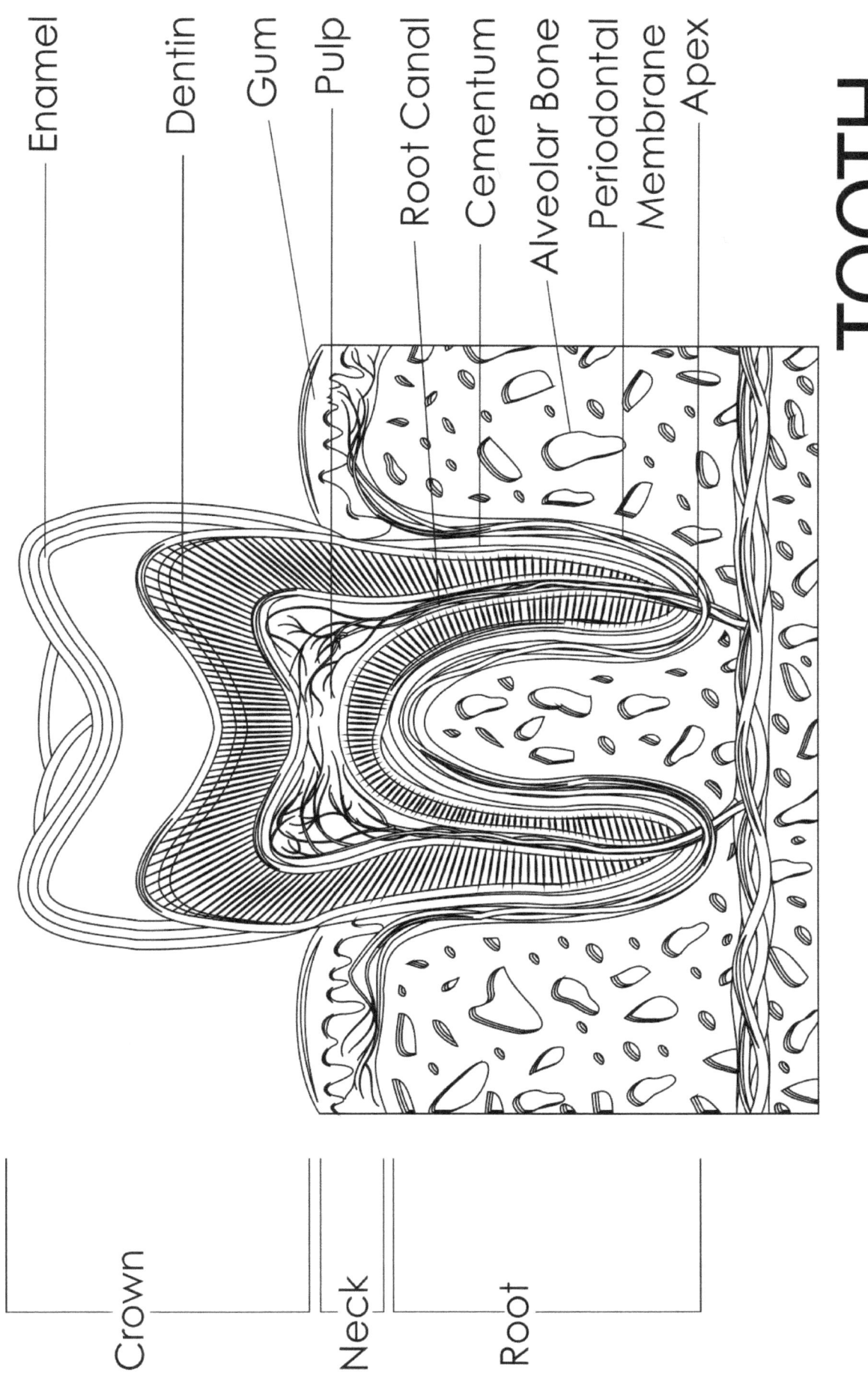

Enamel

Dentin

Gum

Pulp

Root Canal

Cementum

Alveolar Bone

Periodontal
Membrane

Apex

TOOTH

Crown

Neck

Root

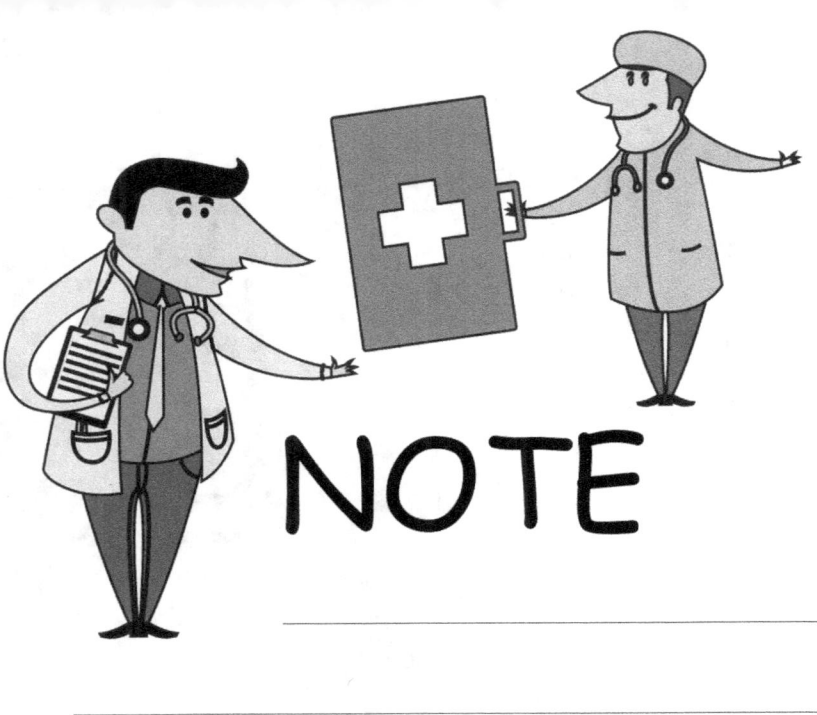

NOTE

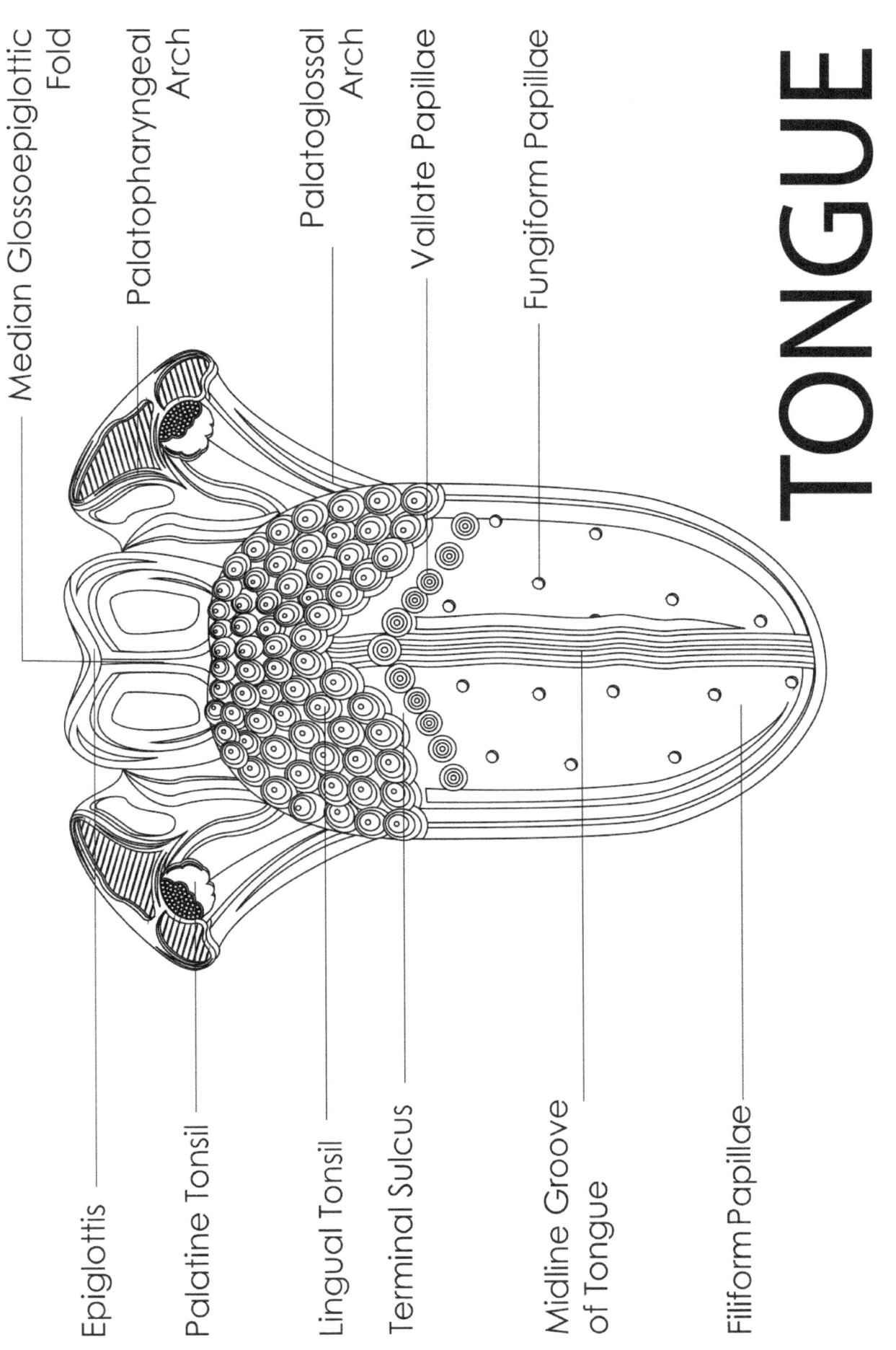

TONGUE

Median Glossoepiglottic Fold

Palatopharyngeal Arch

Palatoglossal Arch

Vallate Papillae

Fungiform Papillae

Epiglottis

Palatine Tonsil

Lingual Tonsil

Terminal Sulcus

Midline Groove of Tongue

Filiform Papillae

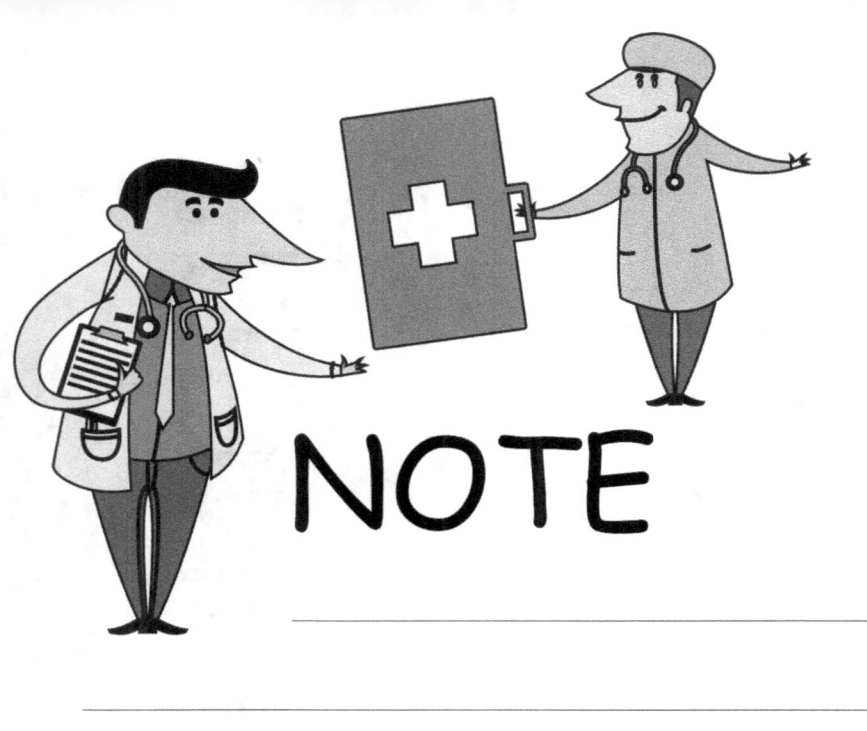

NOTE

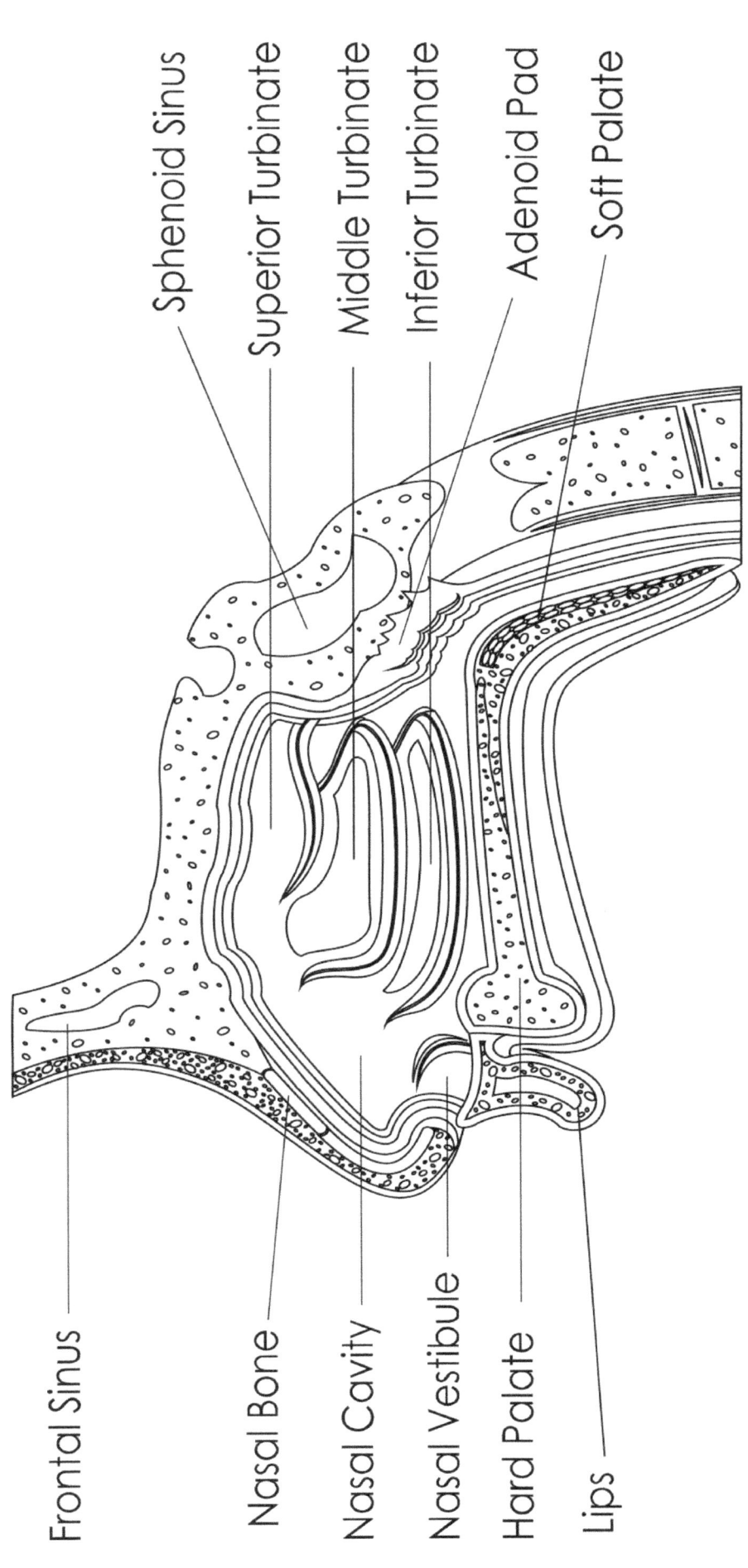

Frontal Sinus

Nasal Bone

Nasal Cavity

Nasal Vestibule

Hard Palate

Lips

Sphenoid Sinus

Superior Turbinate

Middle Turbinate

Inferior Turbinate

Adenoid Pad

Soft Palate

NOSE

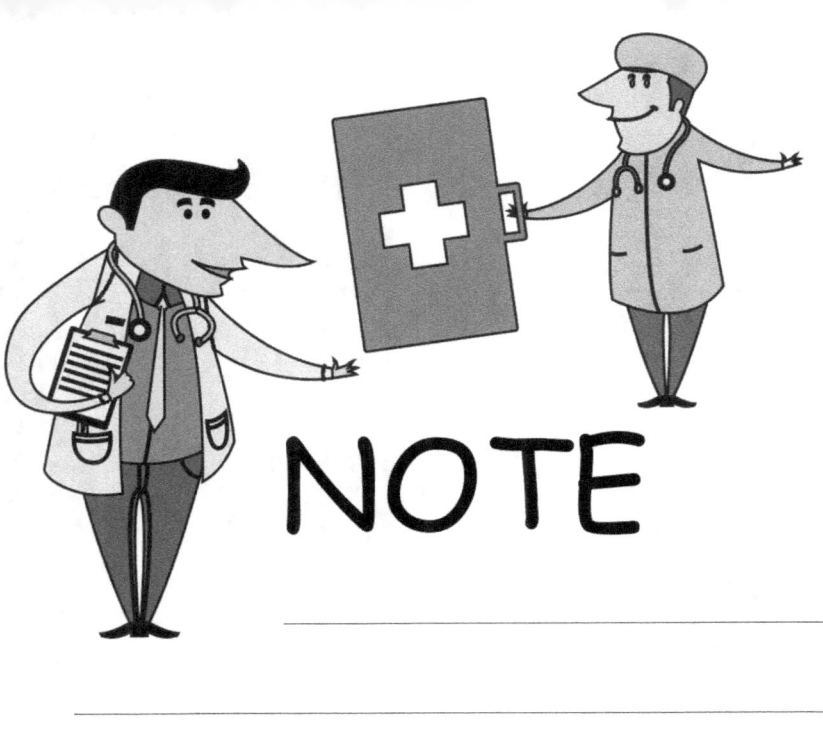

NOTE

THROAT

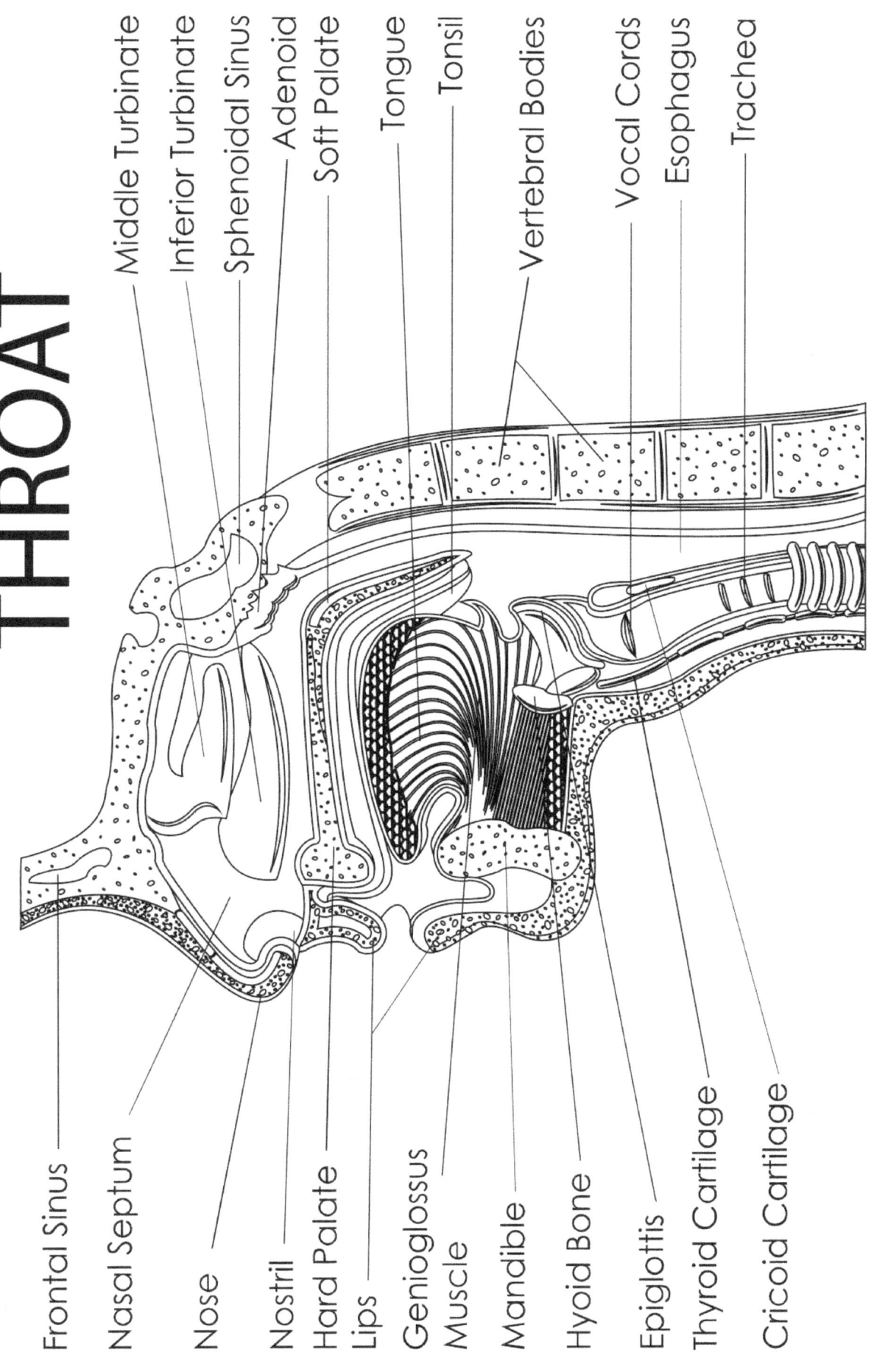

Frontal Sinus
Nasal Septum
Nose
Nostril
Hard Palate
Lips
Genioglossus
Muscle
Mandible
Hyoid Bone
Epiglottis
Thyroid Cartilage
Cricoid Cartilage

Middle Turbinate
Inferior Turbinate
Sphenoidal Sinus
Adenoid
Soft Palate
Tongue
Tonsil
Vertebral Bodies
Vocal Cords
Esophagus
Trachea

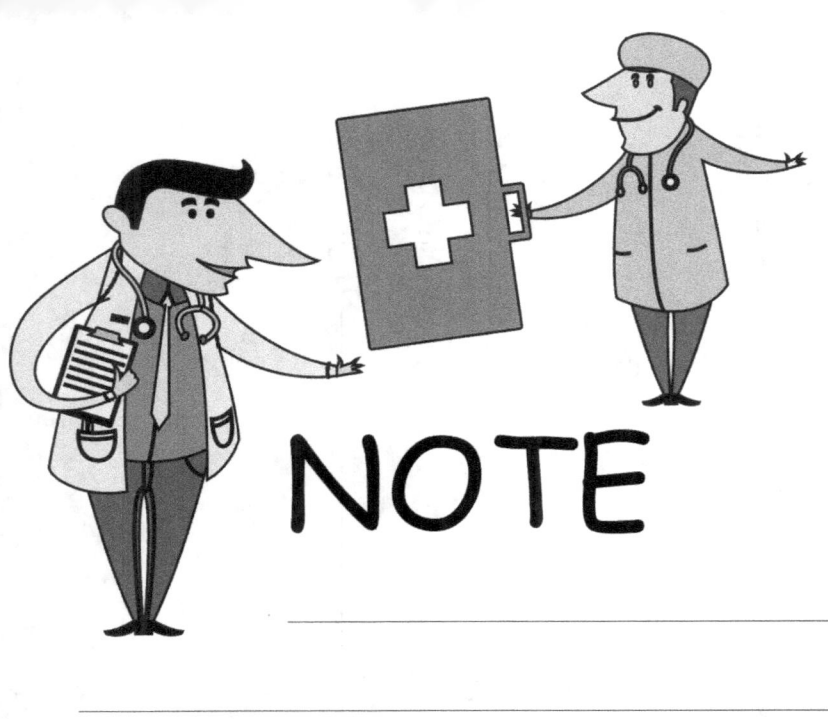

NOTE

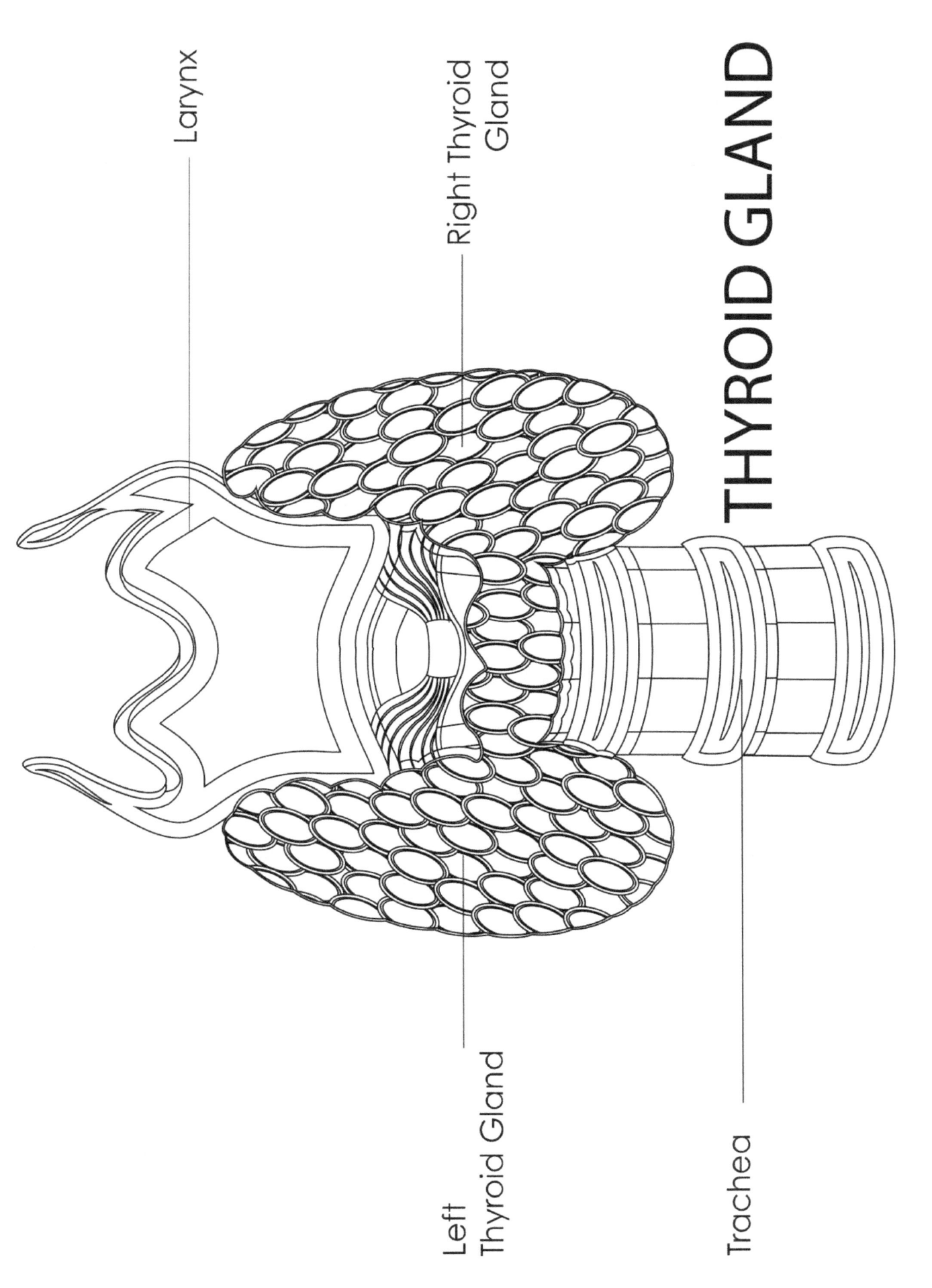

Larynx

Right Thyroid
Gland

Left
Thyroid Gland

Trachea

THYROID GLAND

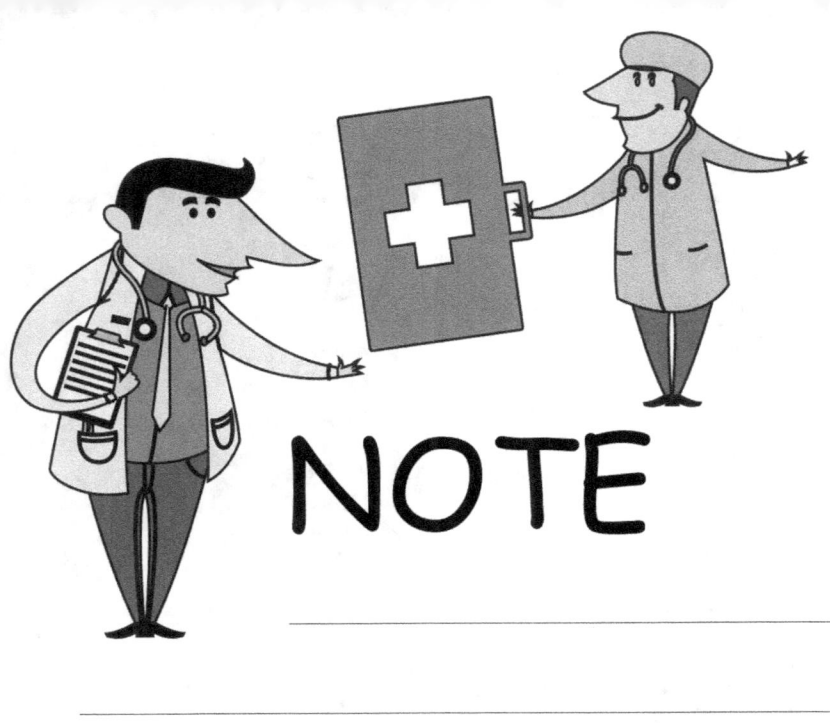

NOTE

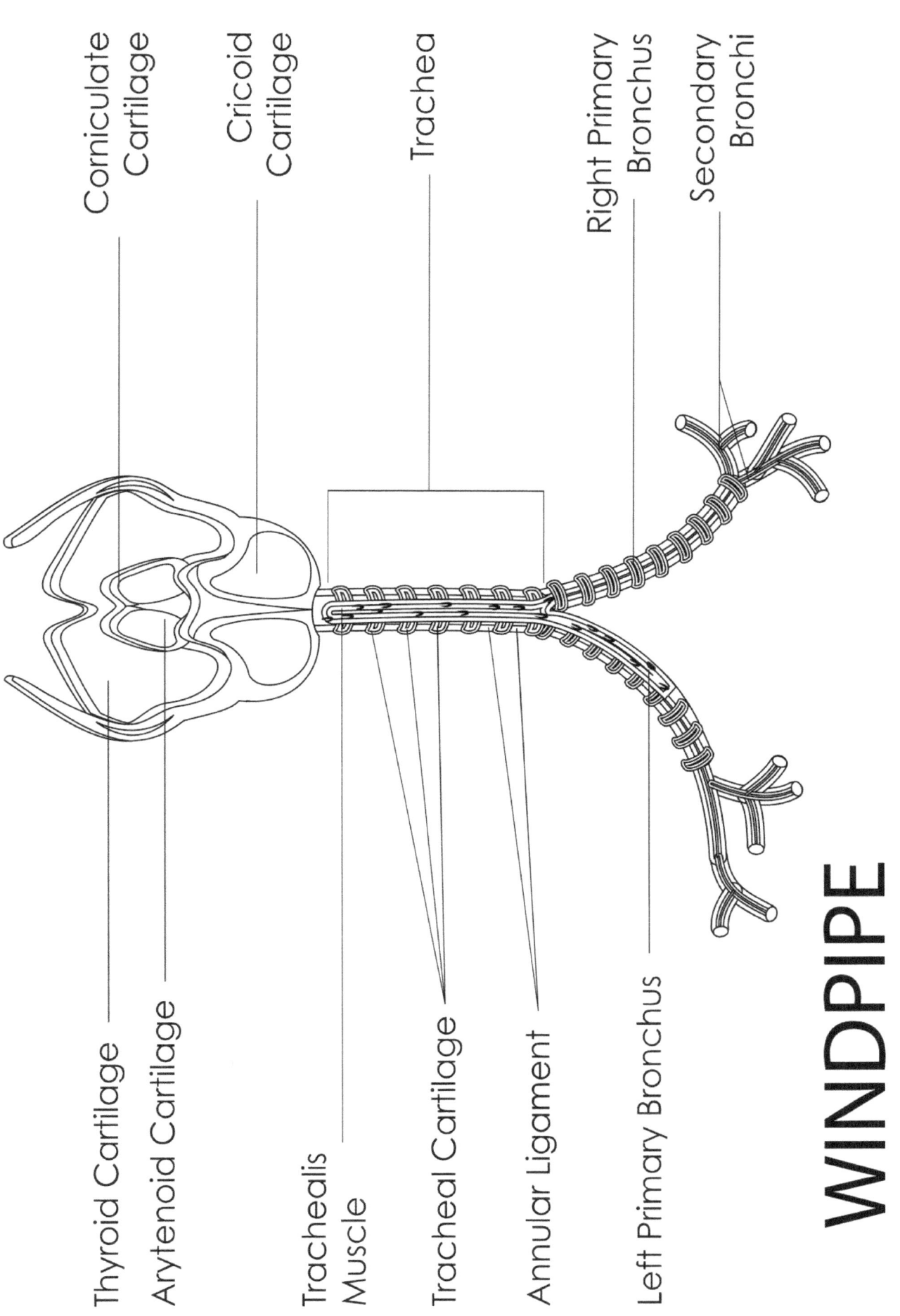

Corniculate Cartilage

Cricoid Cartilage

Trachea

Right Primary Bronchus

Secondary Bronchi

Thyroid Cartilage

Arytenoid Cartilage

Trachealis Muscle

Tracheal Cartilage

Annular Ligament

Left Primary Bronchus

WINDPIPE

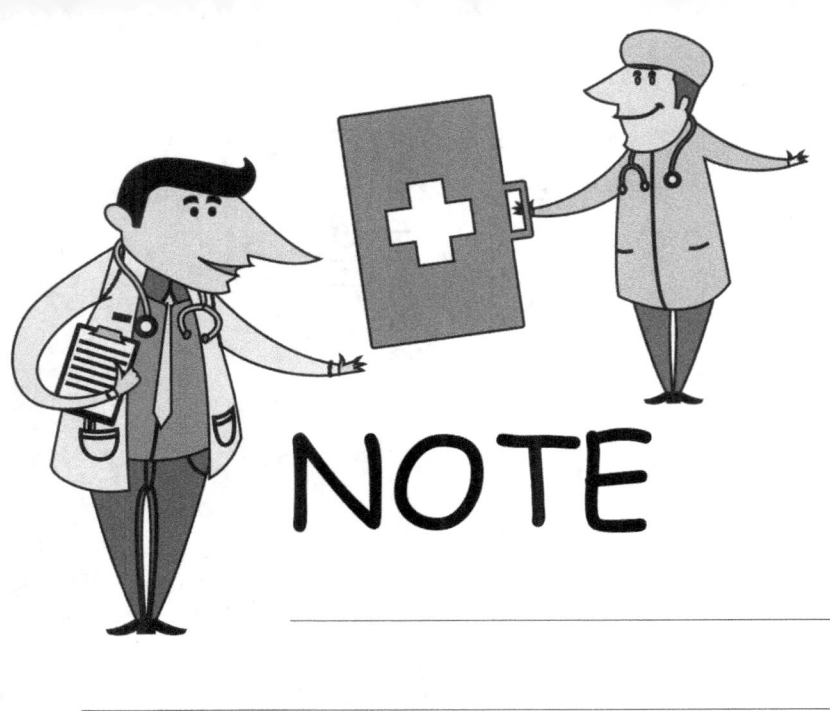

NOTE

LARYNX

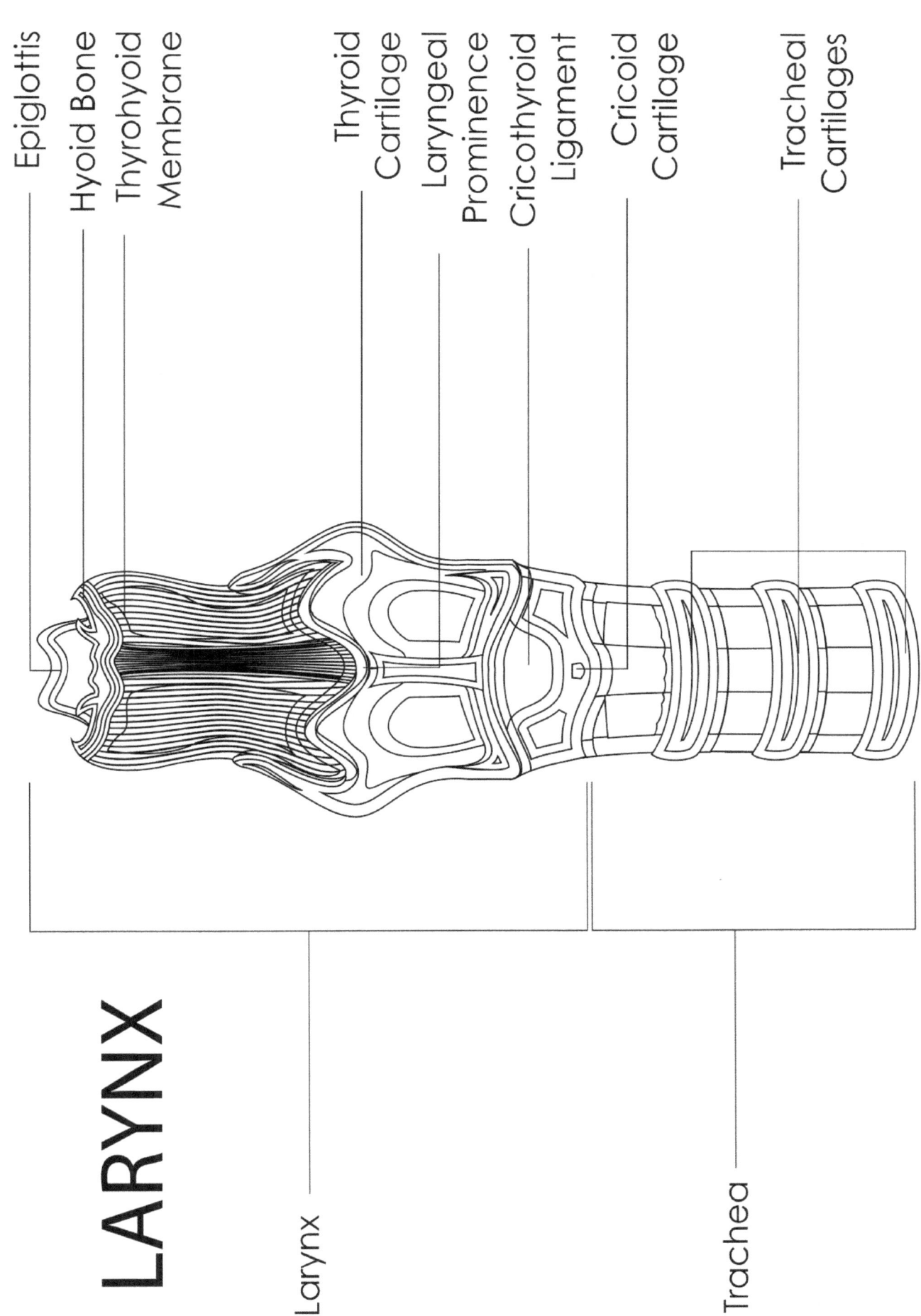

Epiglottis

Hyoid Bone

Thyrohyoid
Membrane

Thyroid
Cartilage

Laryngeal
Prominence

Cricothyroid
Ligament

Cricoid
Cartilage

Tracheal
Cartilages

Larynx

Trachea

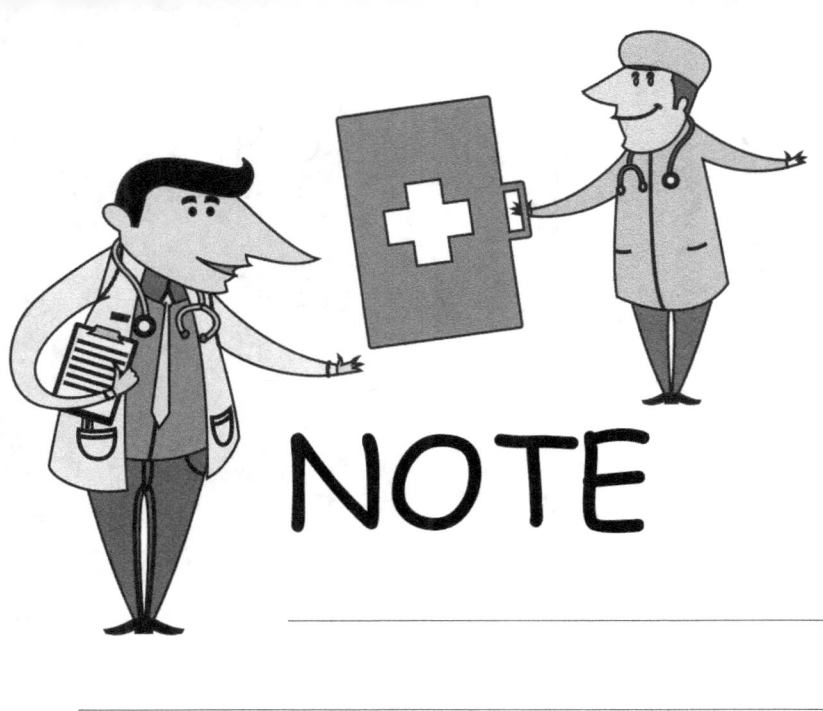

NOTE

EAR

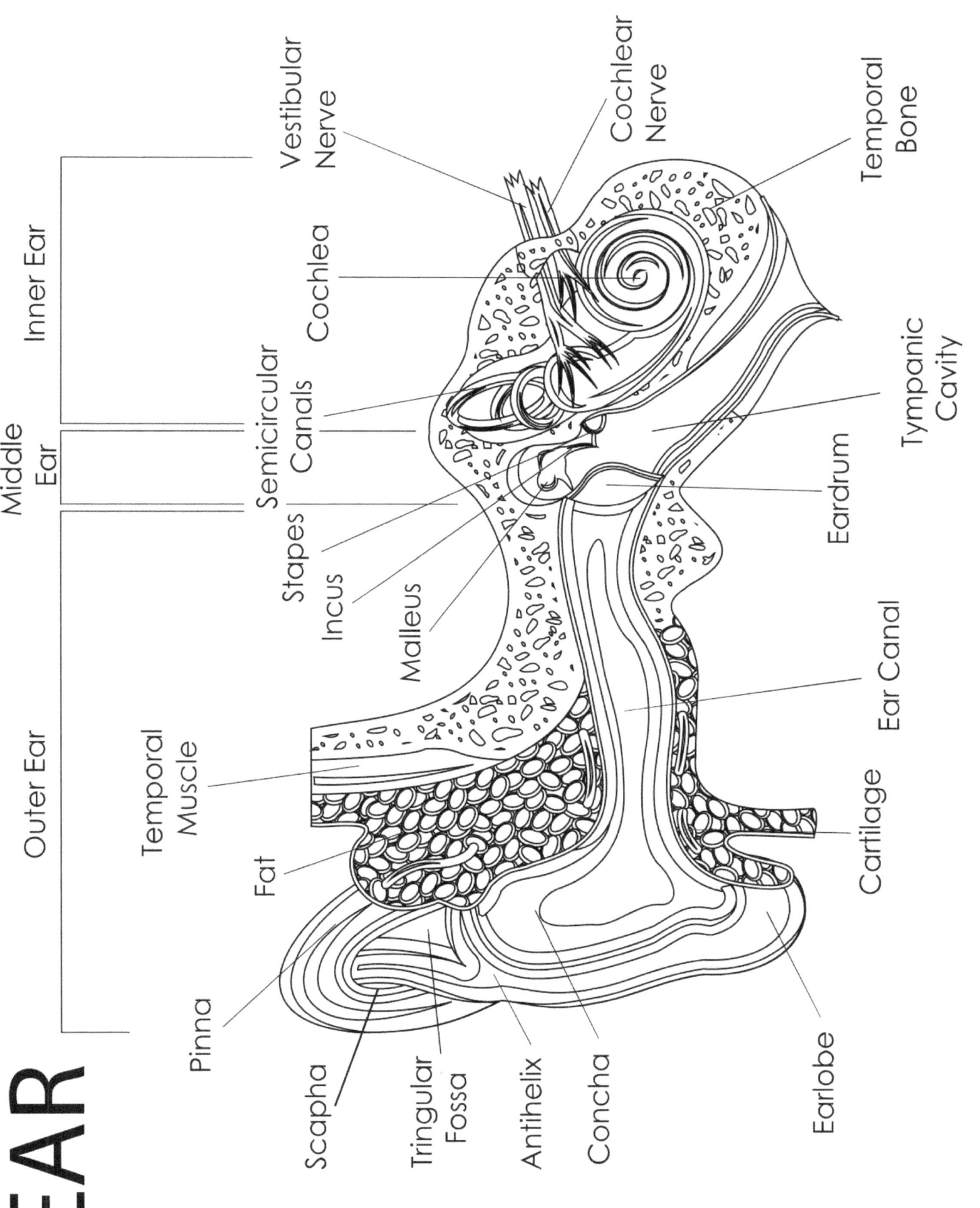

Outer Ear

Middle Ear

Inner Ear

Vestibular Nerve

Cochlear Nerve

Temporal Bone

Cochlea

Semicircular Canals

Stapes

Incus

Malleus

Tympanic Cavity

Eardrum

Temporal Muscle

Fat

Ear Canal

Cartilage

Pinna

Scapha

Tringular Fossa

Antihelix

Concha

Earlobe

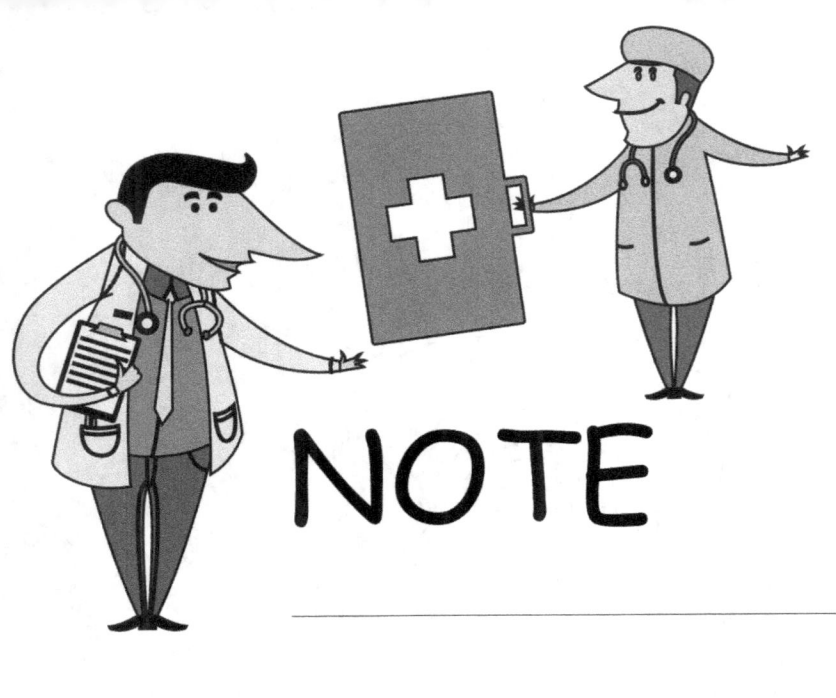

NOTE

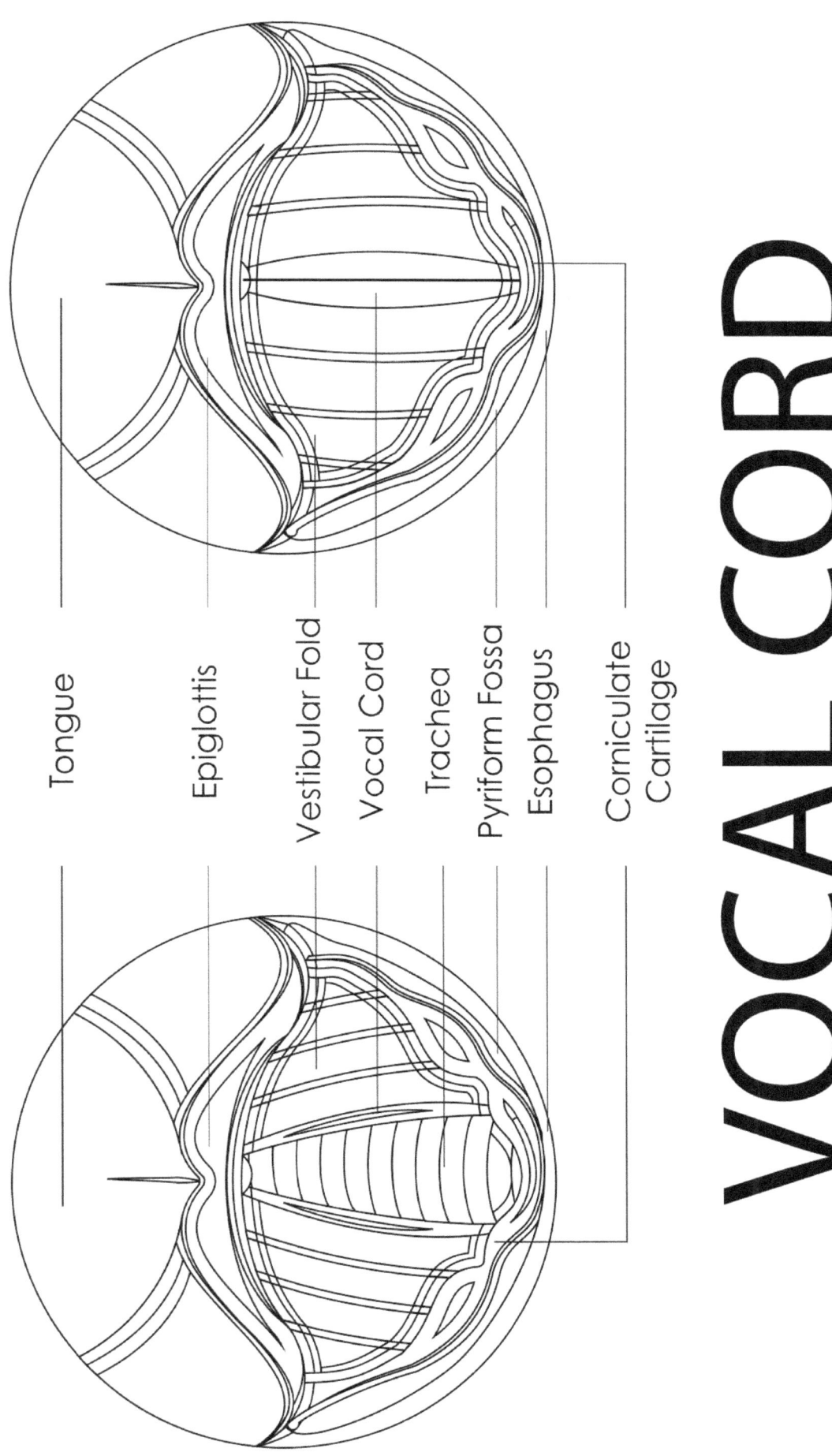

Tongue

Epiglottis

Vestibular Fold

Vocal Cord

Trachea

Pyriform Fossa

Esophagus

Corniculate
Cartilage

VOCAL CORD

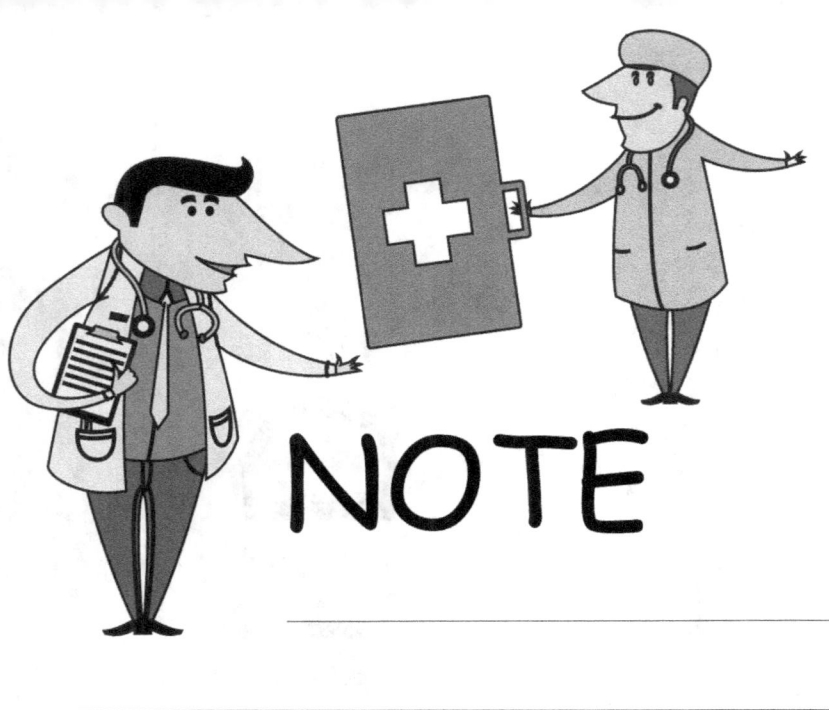

NOTE

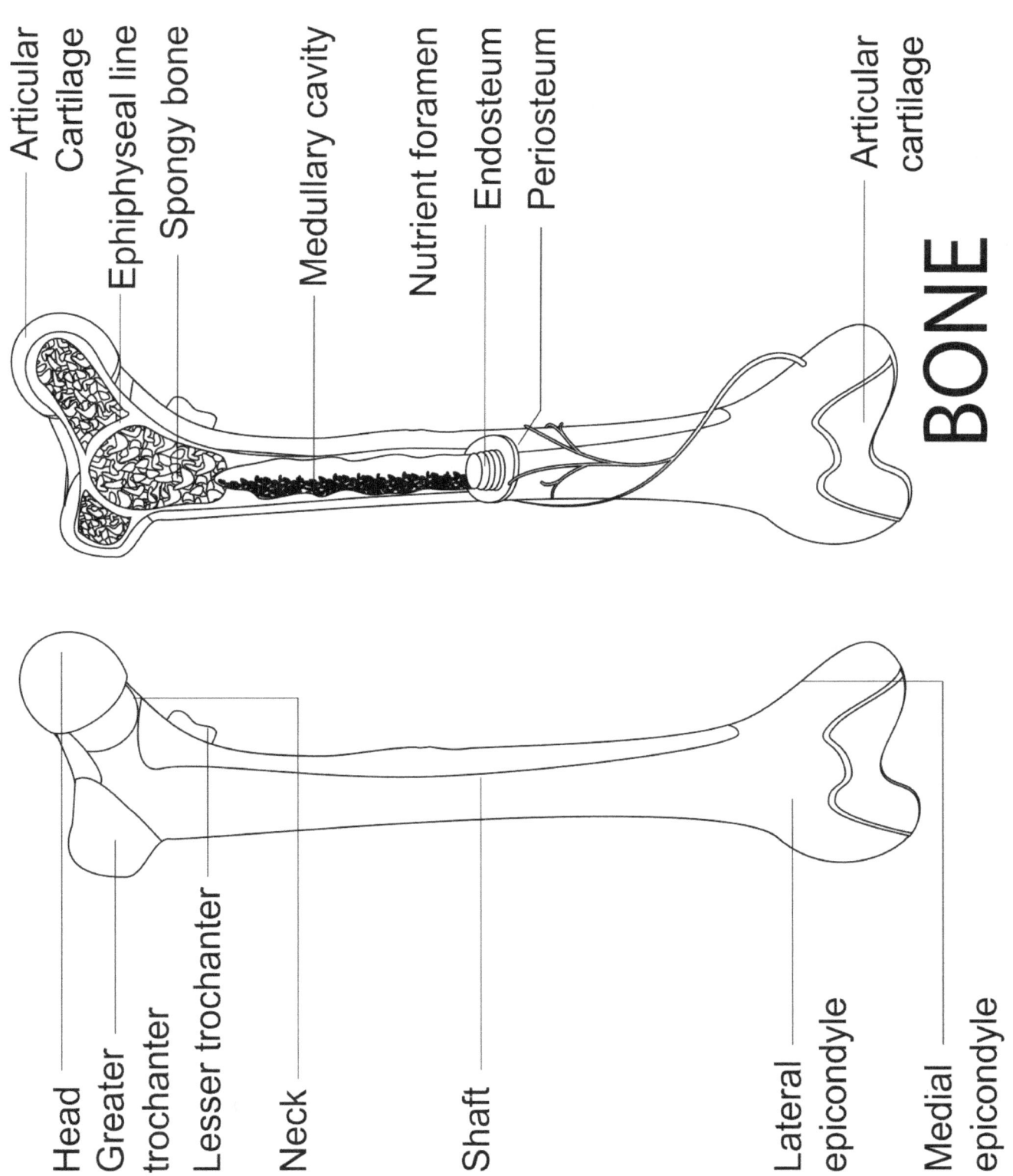

Articular
Cartilage

Ephiphyseal line

Spongy bone

Medullary cavity

Nutrient foramen

Endosteum

Periosteum

Articular
cartilage

BONE

Head

Greater
trochanter

Lesser trochanter

Neck

Shaft

Lateral
epicondyle

Medial
epicondyle

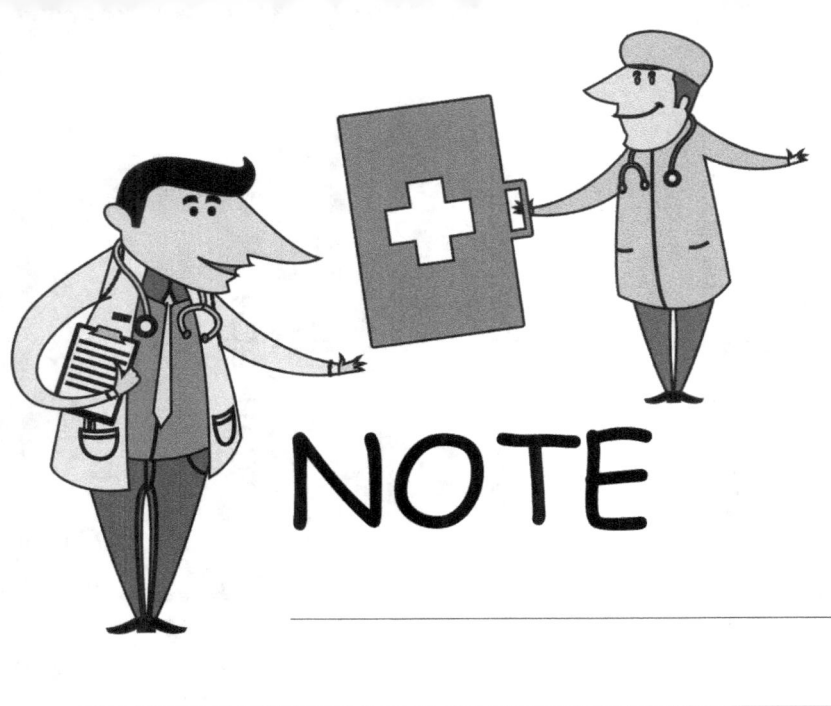

NOTE

TEETH

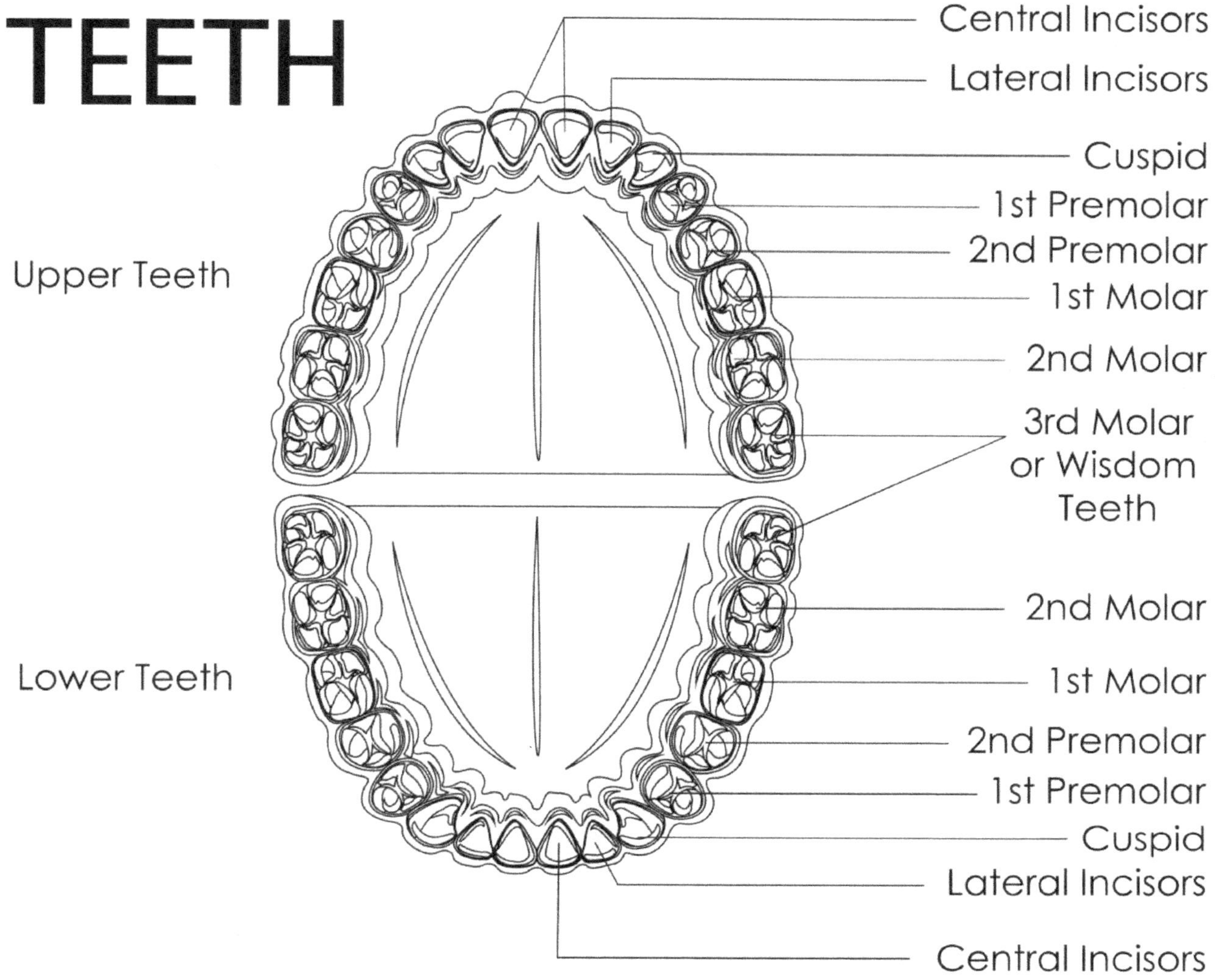

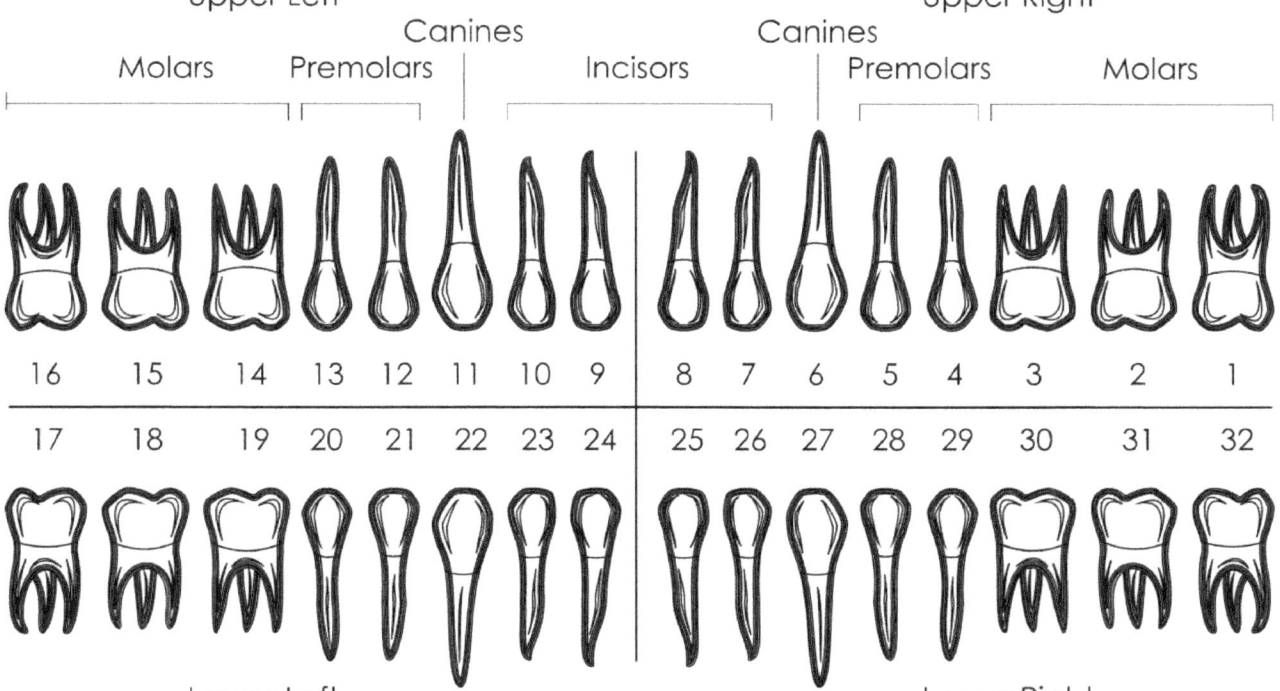

Upper Teeth

- Central Incisors
- Lateral Incisors
- Cuspid
- 1st Premolar
- 2nd Premolar
- 1st Molar
- 2nd Molar
- 3rd Molar or Wisdom Teeth

Lower Teeth

- 2nd Molar
- 1st Molar
- 2nd Premolar
- 1st Premolar
- Cuspid
- Lateral Incisors
- Central Incisors

Upper Left

Upper Right

Molars   Premolars   Canines   Incisors   Canines   Premolars   Molars

16 15 14 13 12 11 10 9 8 7 6 5 4 3 2 1

17 18 19 20 21 22 23 24 25 26 27 28 29 30 31 32

Lower Left

Lower Right

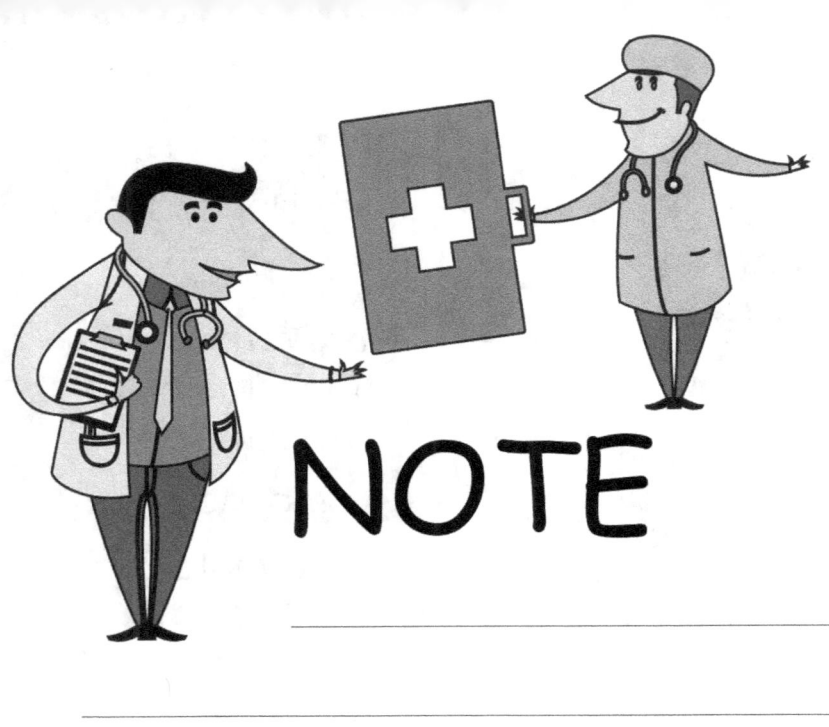

NOTE

_____

_____

_____

_____

_____

_____

_____

_____

_____

_____

_____

_____

_____

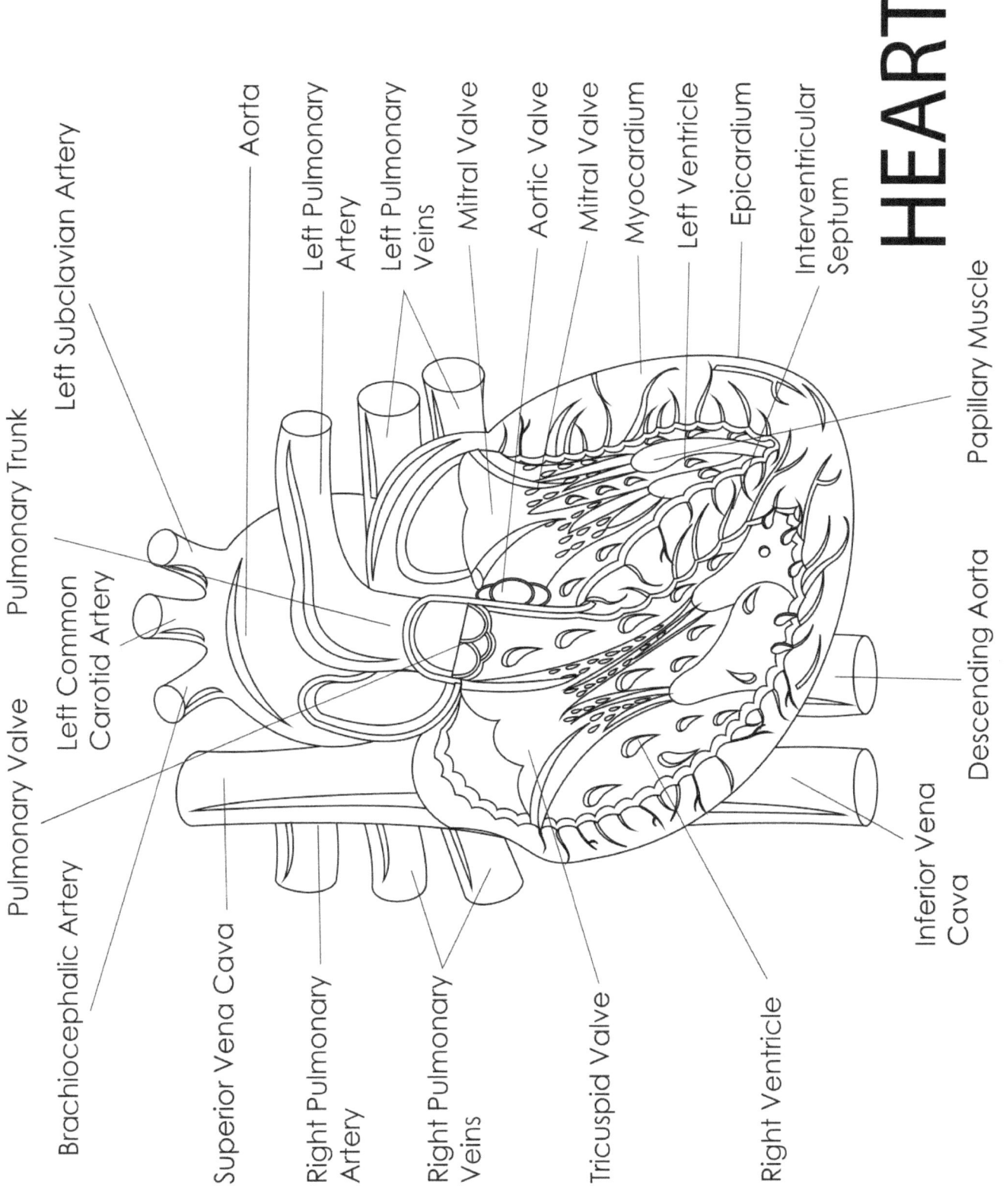

Brachiocephalic Artery

Pulmonary Valve

Pulmonary Trunk

Left Common
Carotid Artery

Left Subclavian Artery

Aorta

Left Pulmonary
Artery

Left Pulmonary
Veins

Mitral Valve

Aortic Valve

Mitral Valve

Myocardium

Left Ventricle

Epicardium

Interventricular
Septum

Superior Vena Cava

Right Pulmonary
Artery

Right Pulmonary
Veins

Tricuspid Valve

Right Ventricle

Inferior Vena
Cava

Descending Aorta

Papillary Muscle

HEART

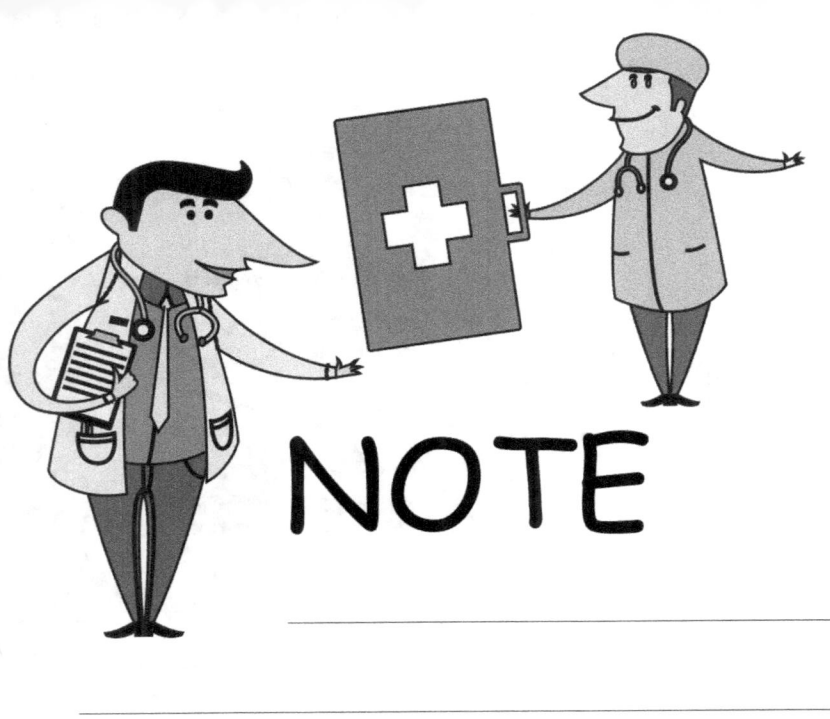

NOTE

LUNGS

Trachea

Bronchioles

Left Main
Stem Bronchus

Bronchi

Left Lobes

Pleura

Pleural Fluid

Left Lung

Right Lung

Right Main
Stem Bronchus

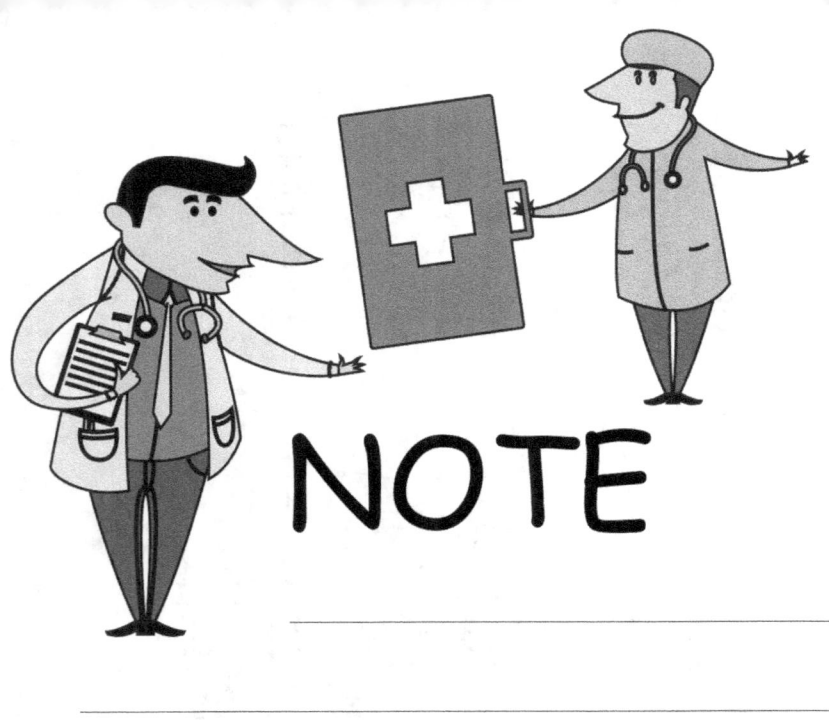

NOTE

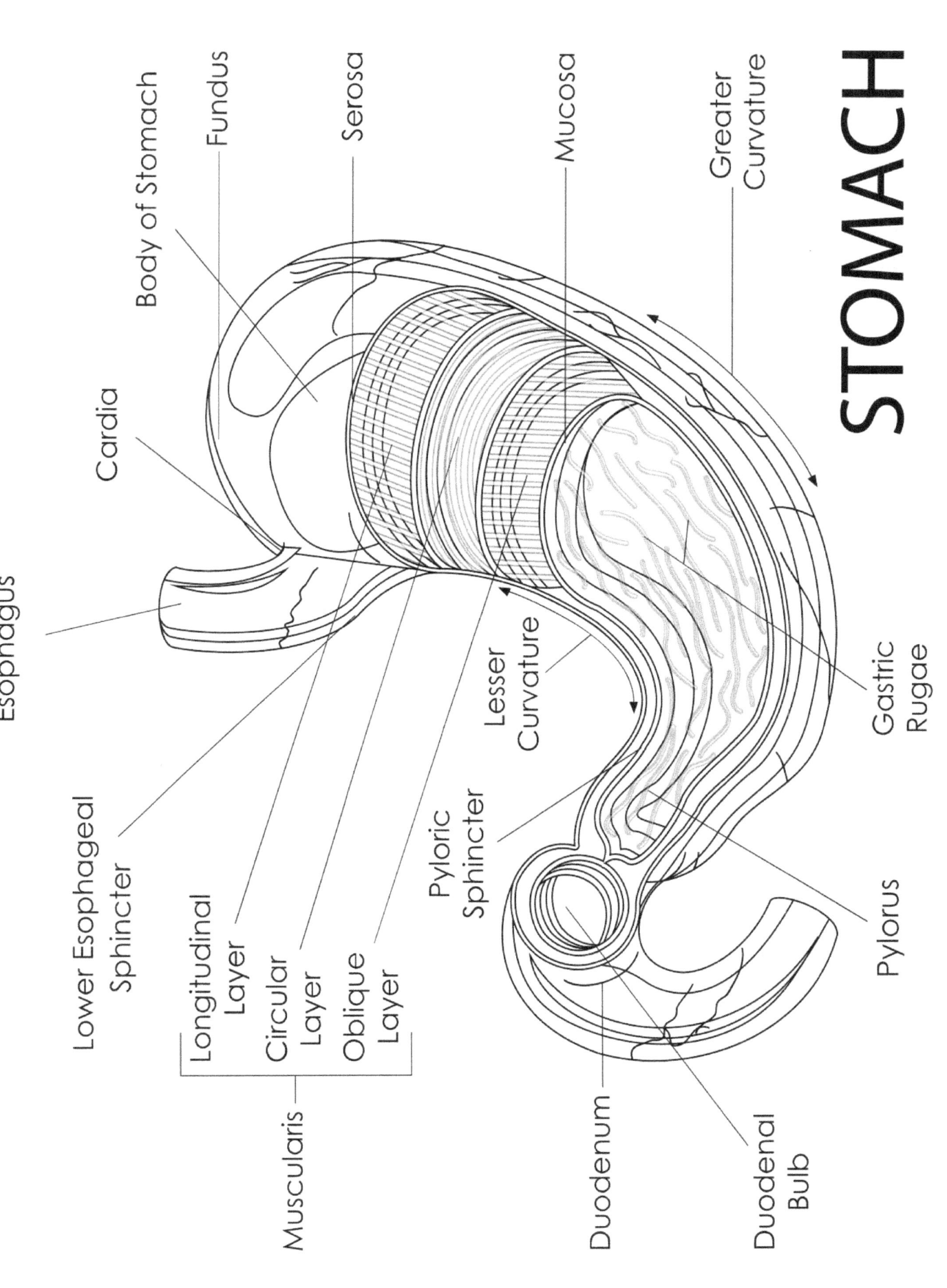

STOMACH

Esophagus

Fundus

Body of Stomach

Cardia

Serosa

Mucosa

Greater Curvature

Lower Esophageal Sphincter

Longitudinal Layer

Circular Layer

Oblique Layer

Muscularis

Lesser Curvature

Pyloric Sphincter

Gastric Rugae

Duodenum

Pylorus

Duodenal Bulb

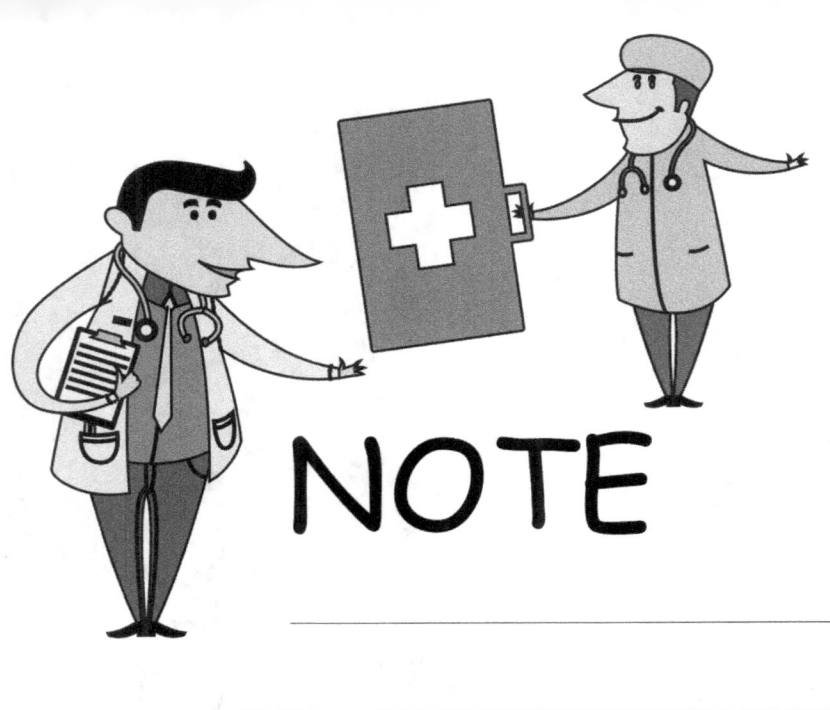

NOTE

_____

_____

_____

_____

_____

_____

_____

_____

_____

_____

_____

_____

_____

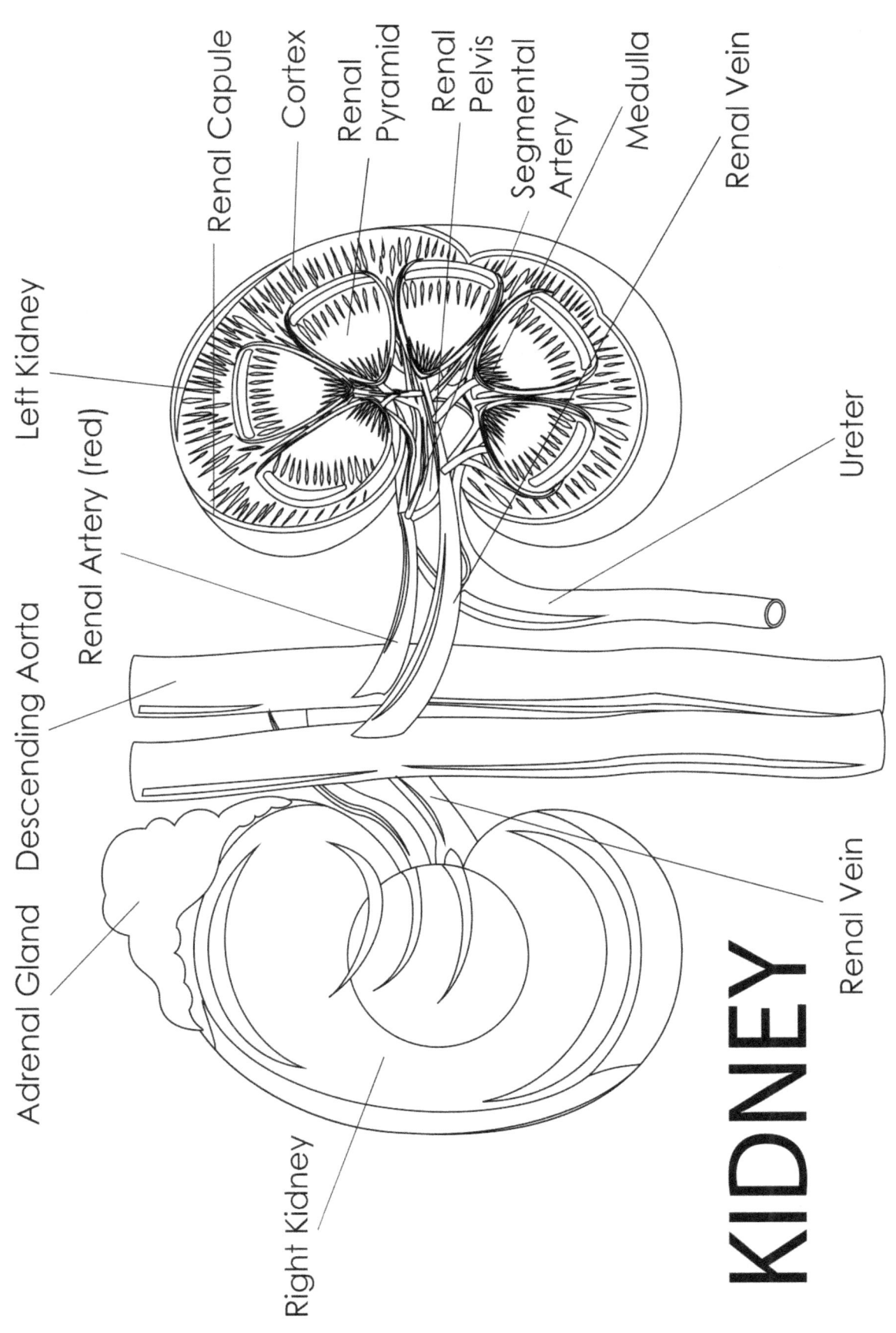

Renal Capule

Cortex

Renal Pyramid

Renal Pelvis

Segmental Artery

Medulla

Renal Vein

Left Kidney

Renal Artery (red)

Adrenal Gland   Descending Aorta

Right Kidney

Ureter

Renal Vein

KIDNEY

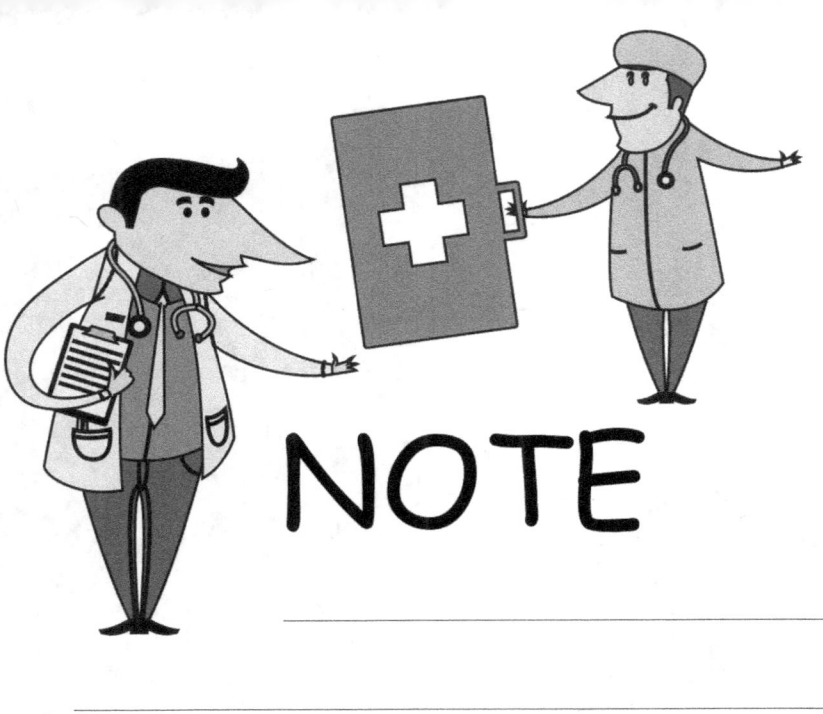

NOTE

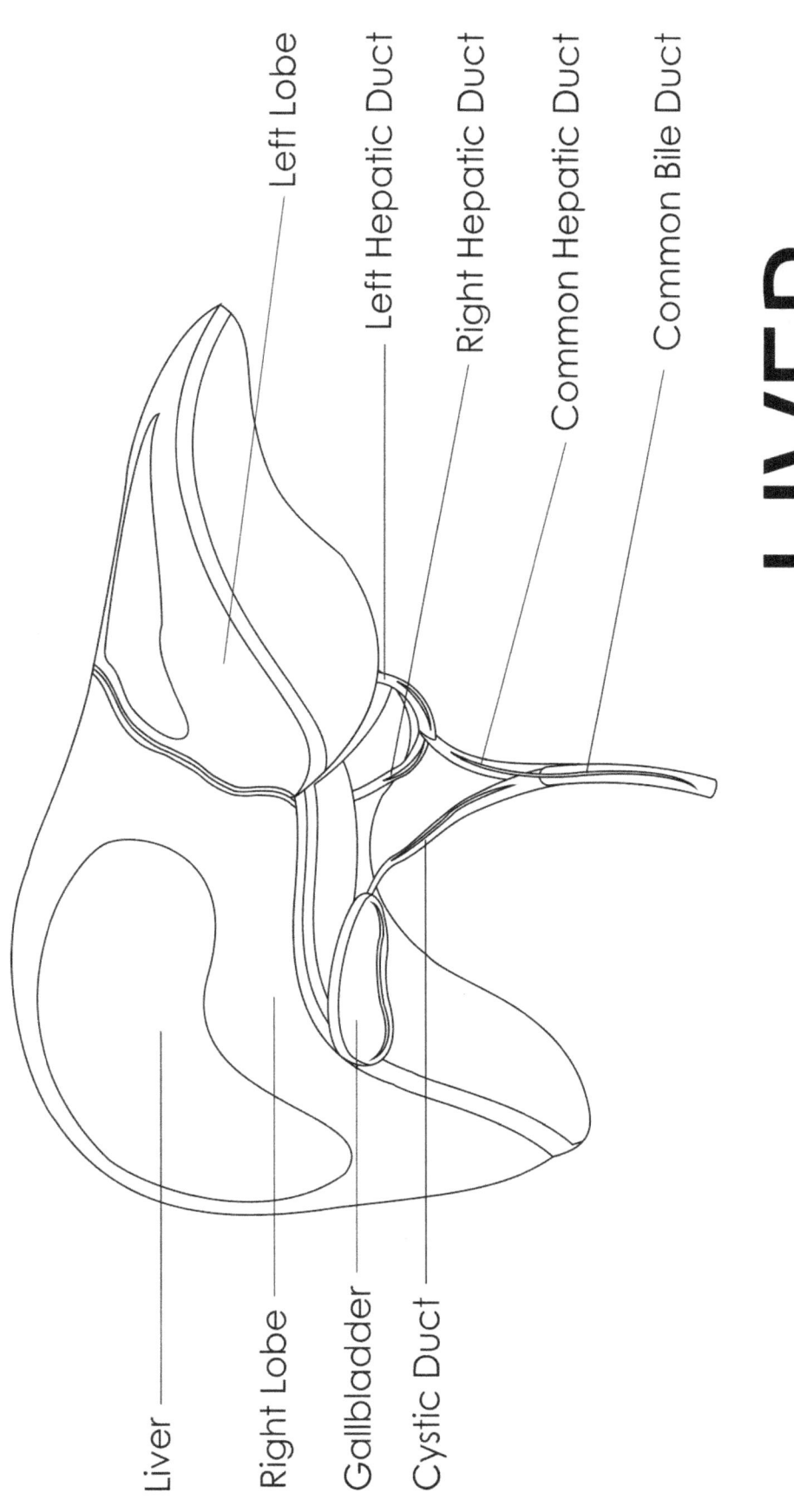

Liver

Right Lobe

Gallbladder

Cystic Duct

Left Lobe

Left Hepatic Duct

Right Hepatic Duct

Common Hepatic Duct

Common Bile Duct

LIVER

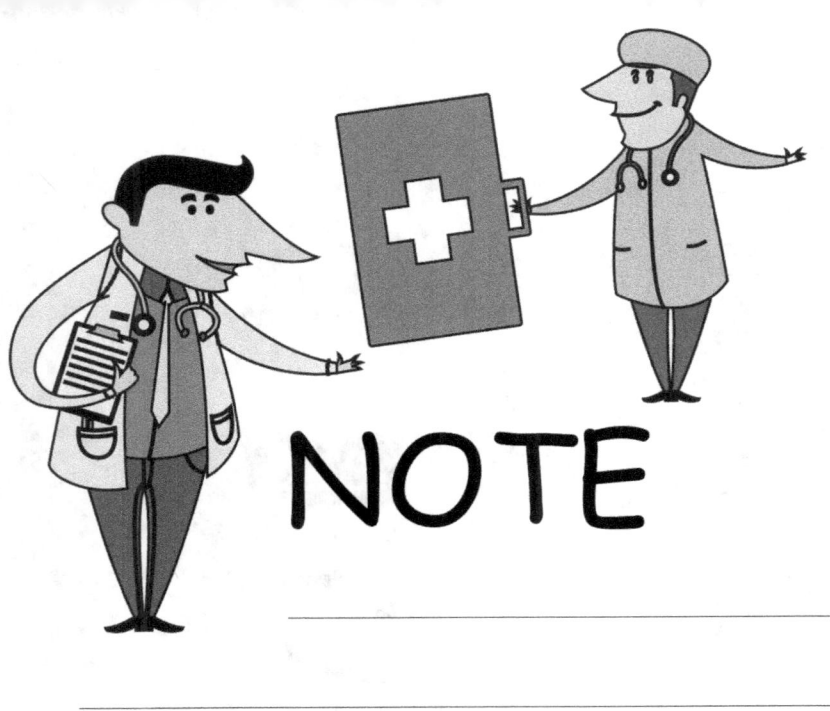

NOTE

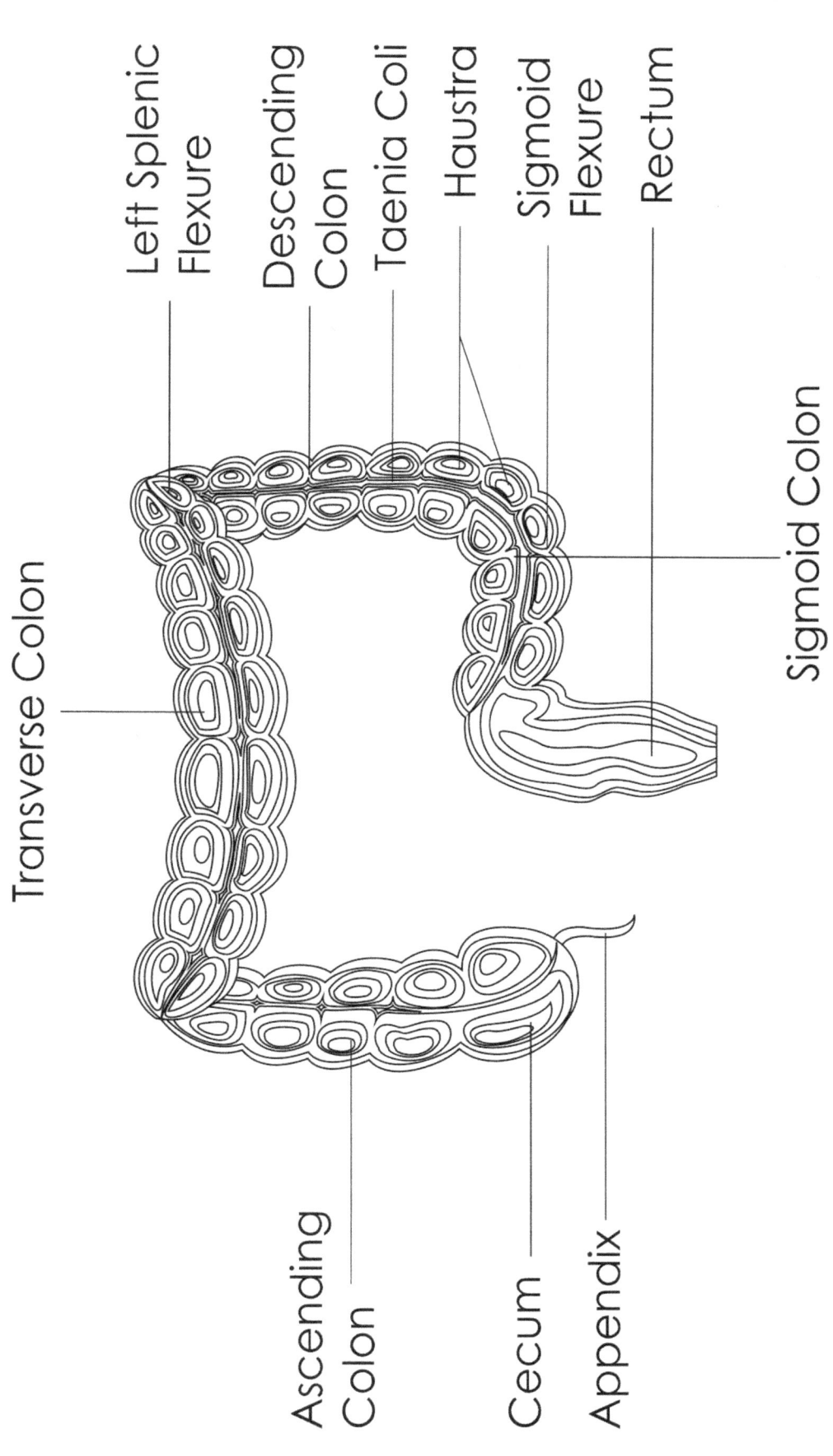

Transverse Colon

Left Splenic Flexure

Descending Colon

Taenia Coli

Haustra

Sigmoid Flexure

Rectum

Sigmoid Colon

Ascending Colon

Cecum

Appendix

LARGE INTESTINE

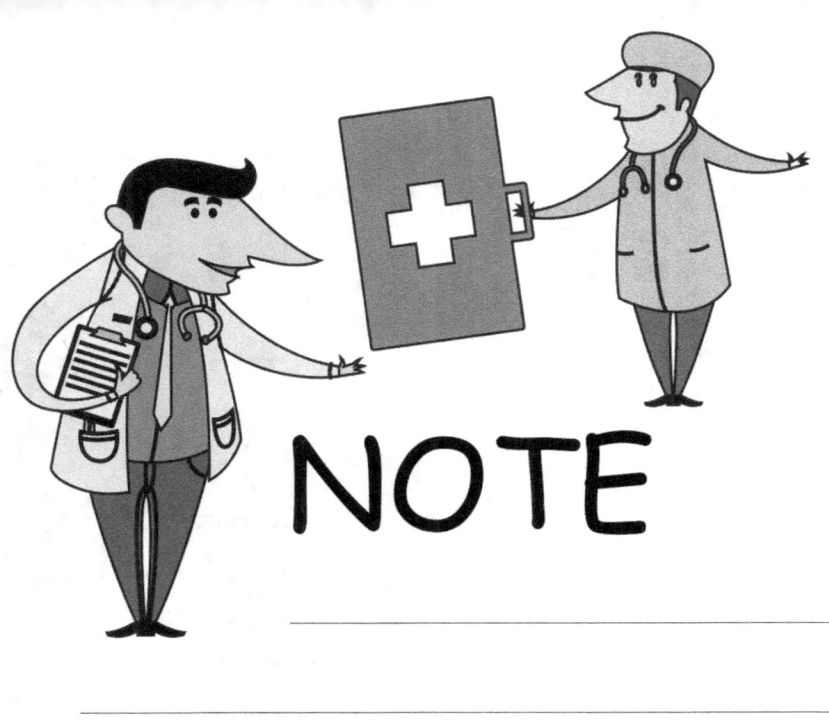

NOTE

_____

_____

_____

_____

_____

_____

_____

_____

_____

_____

_____

_____

_____

_____

_____

FLOW OF BLOOD

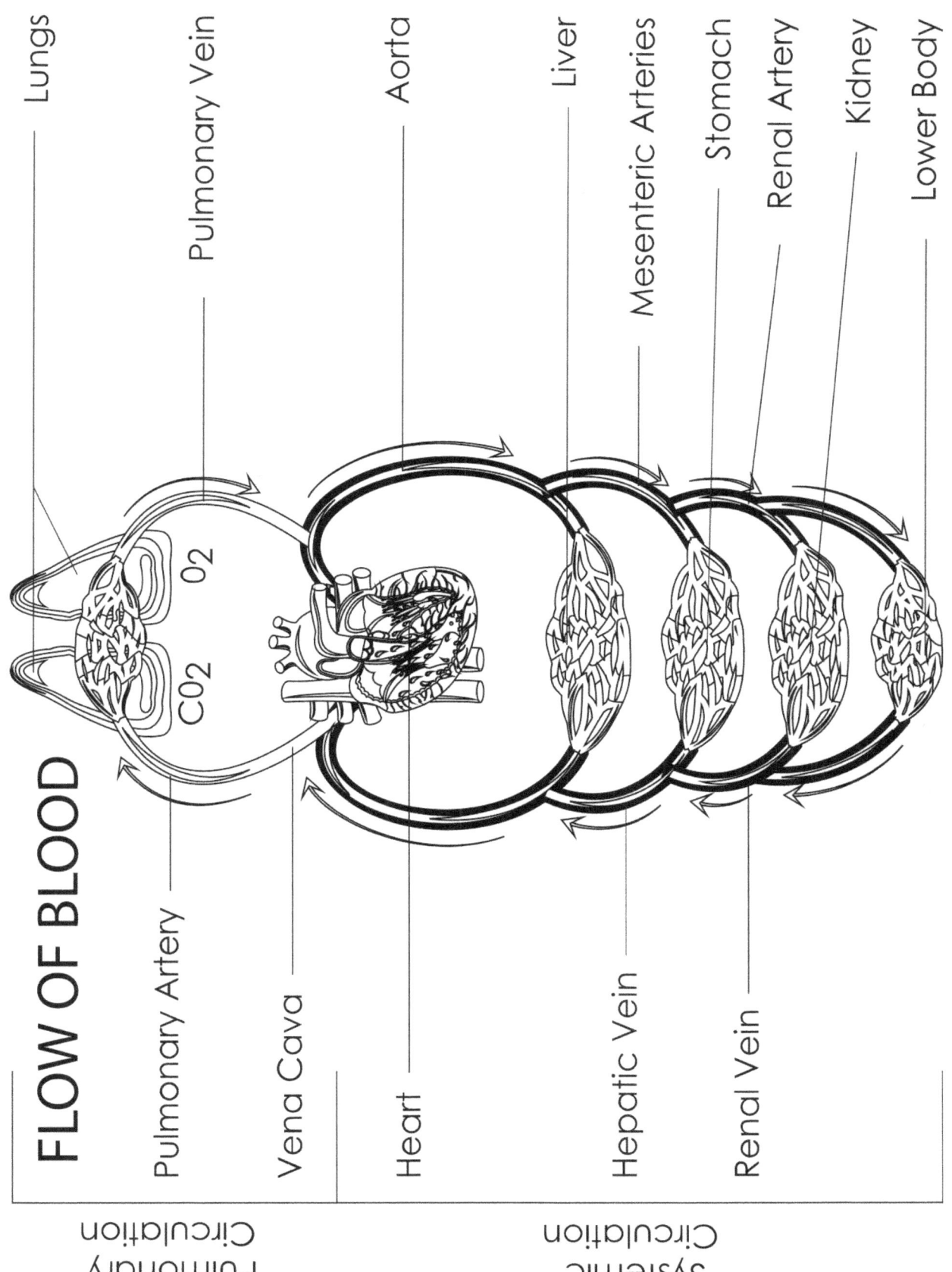

Lungs

Pulmonary Vein

Aorta

Liver

Mesenteric Arteries

Stomach

Renal Artery

Kidney

Lower Body

Pulmonary Artery

Vena Cava

Heart

Hepatic Vein

Renal Vein

O2

CO2

Pulmonary Circulation

Systemic Circulation

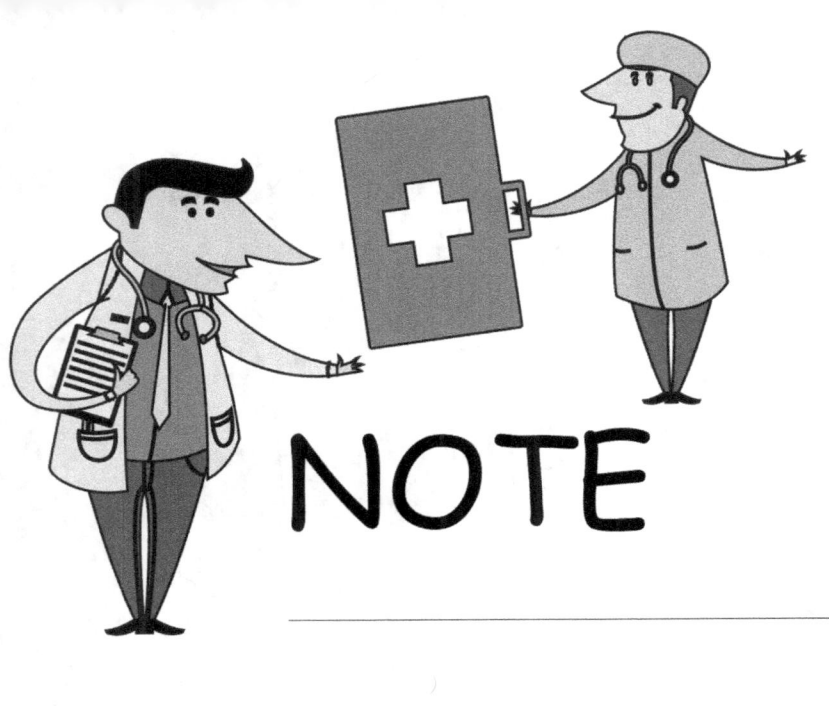

NOTE

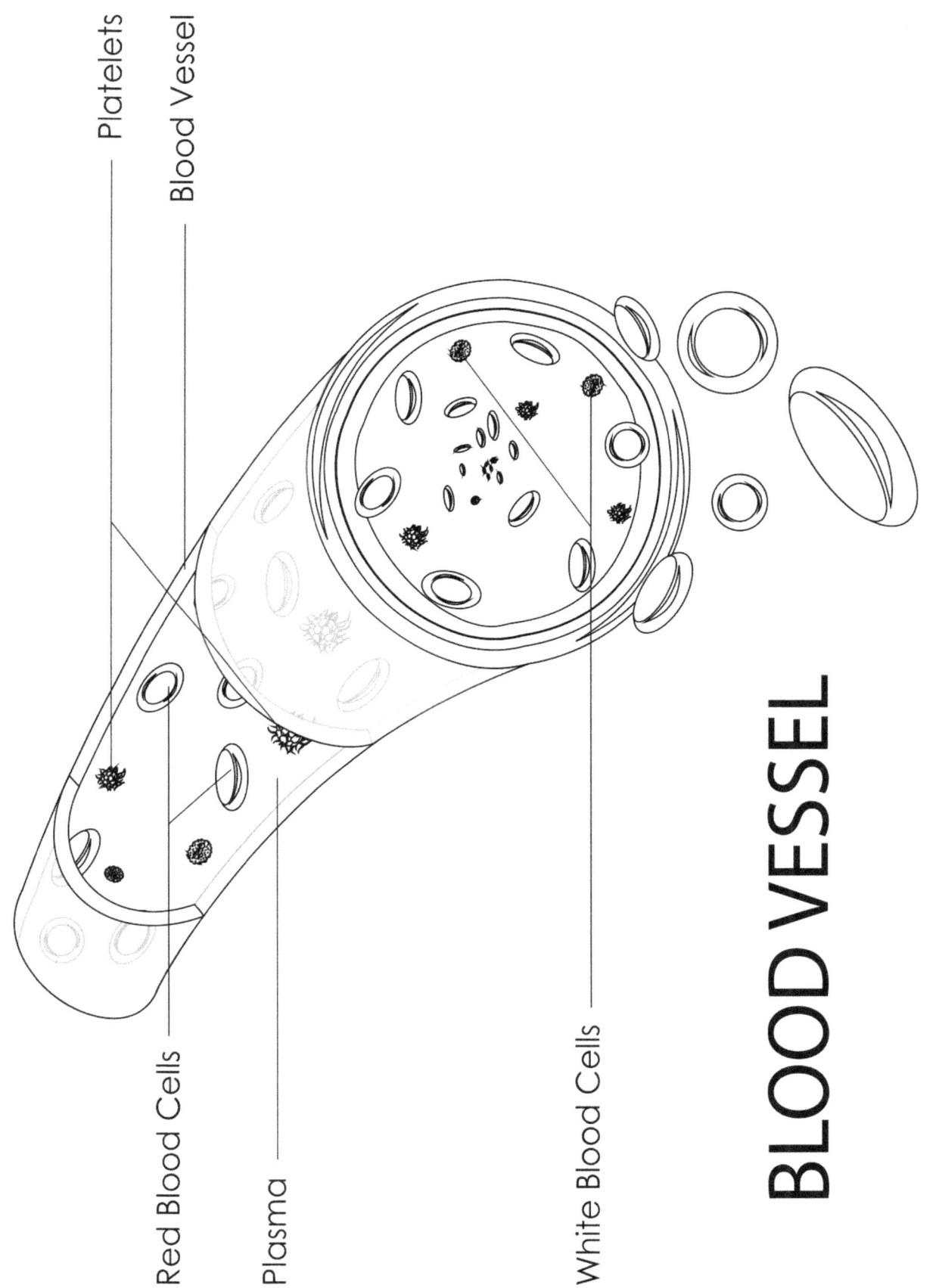

Platelets

Blood Vessel

Red Blood Cells

Plasma

White Blood Cells

BLOOD VESSEL

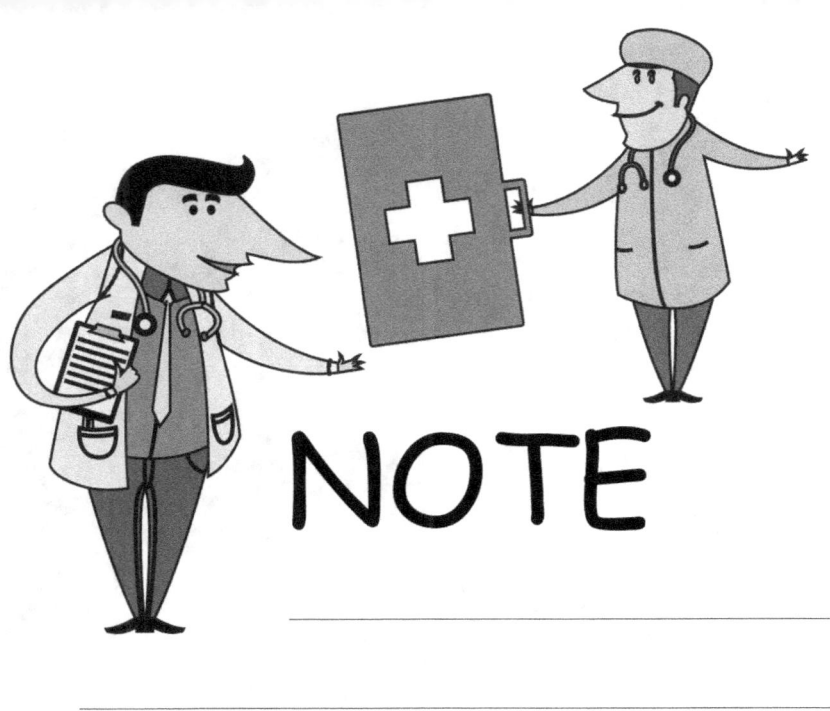

NOTE

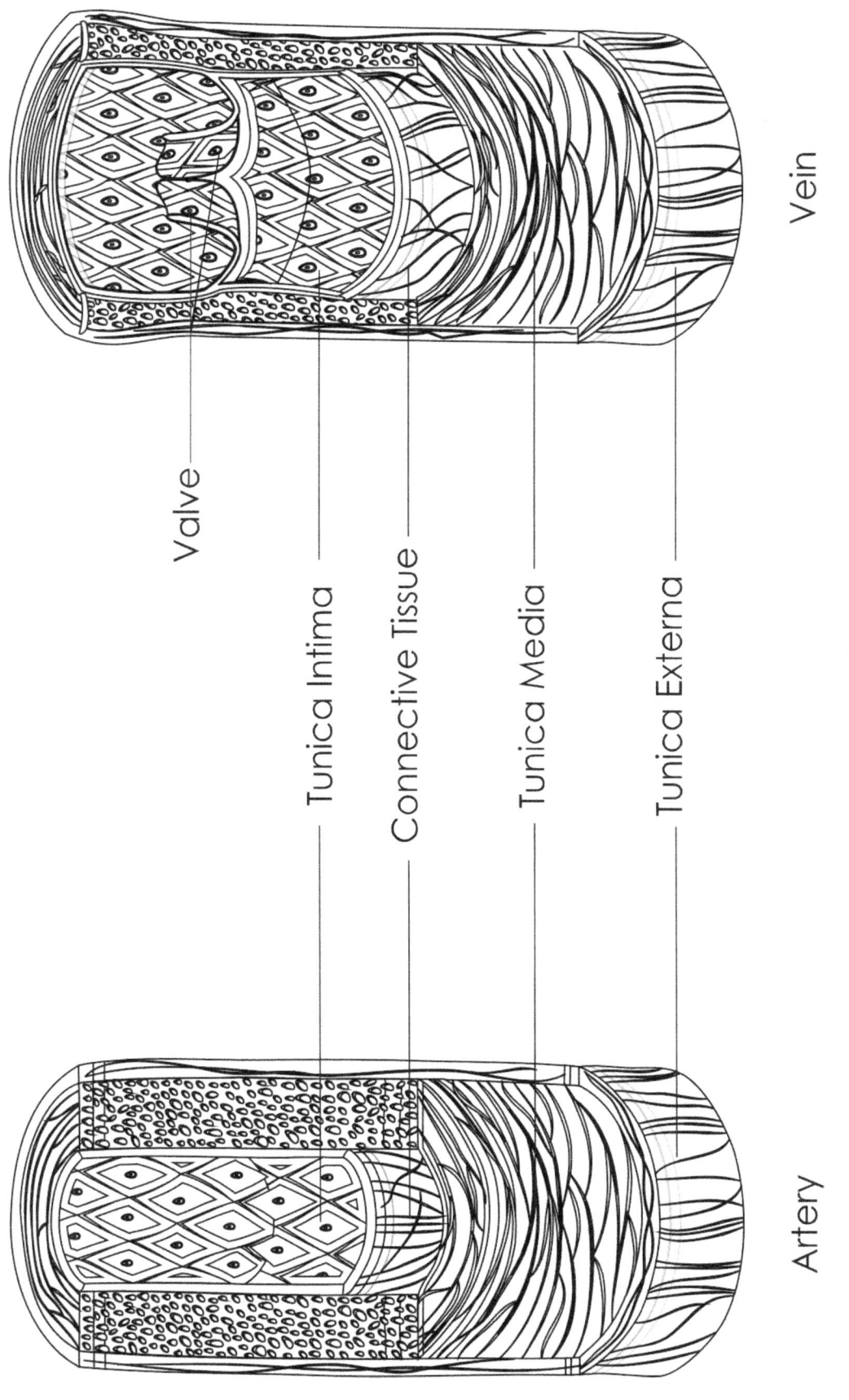

Valve

Tunica Intima

Connective Tissue

Tunica Media

Tunica Externa

Vein

Artery

ARTERY AND VEIN

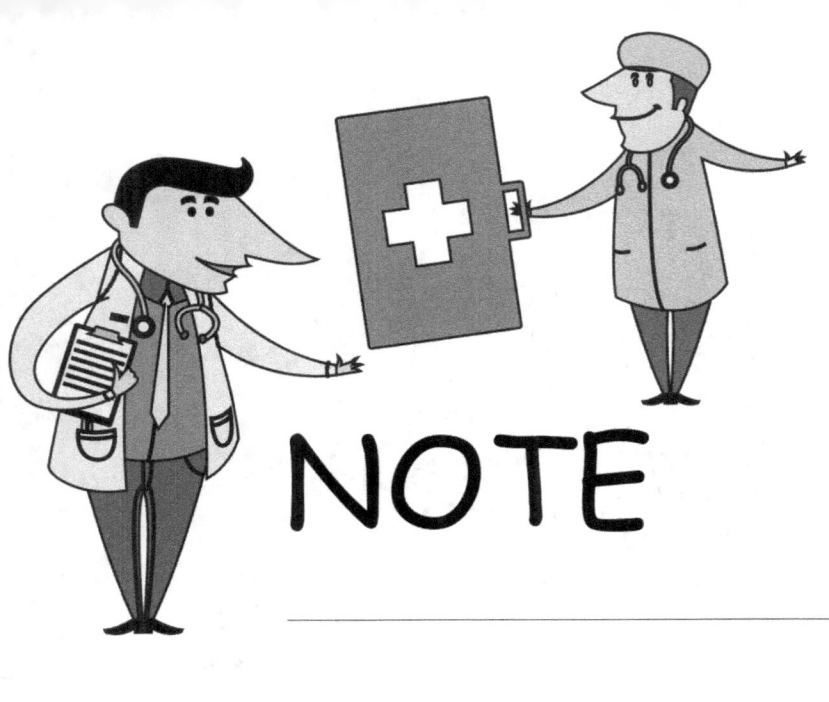

NOTE

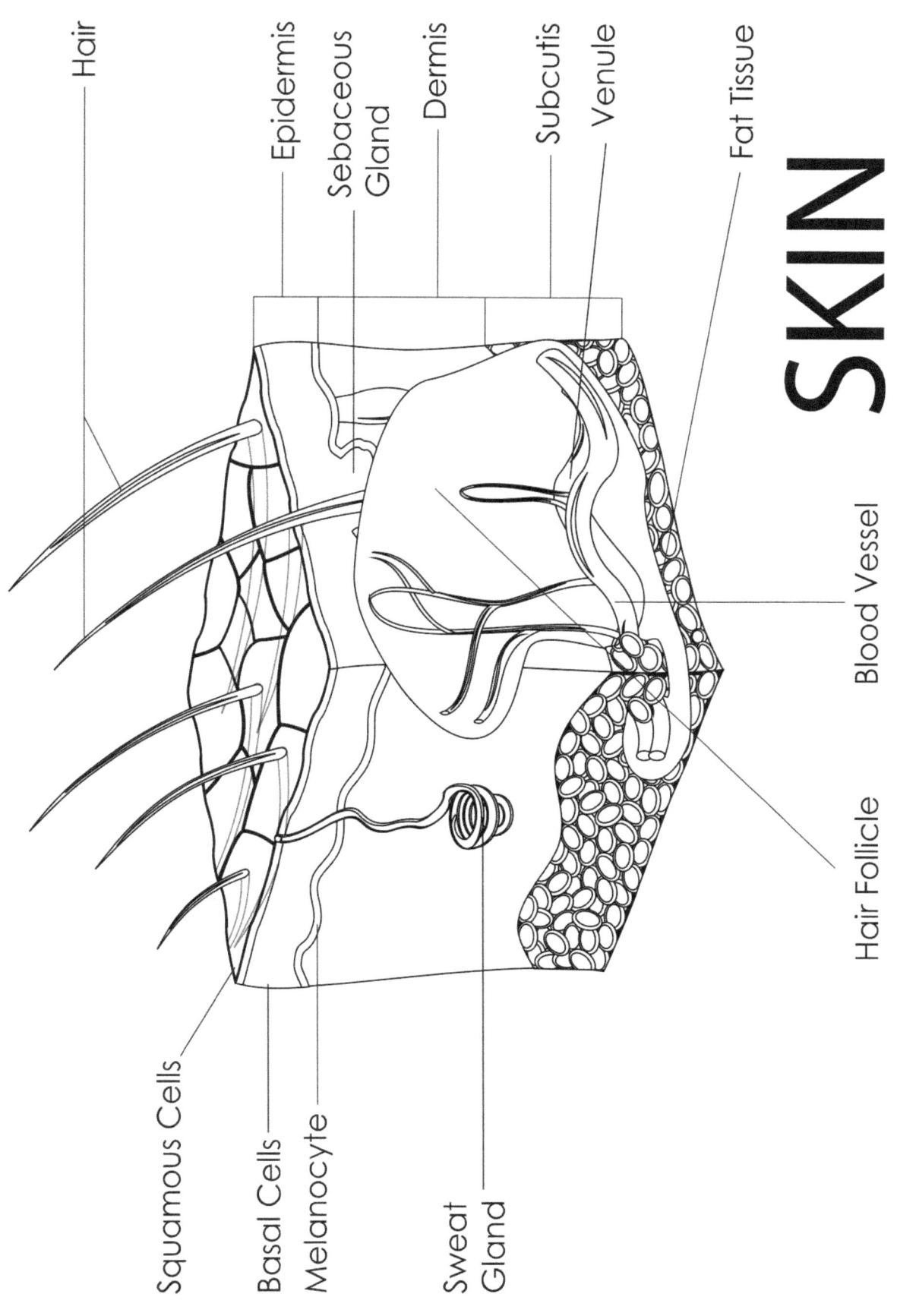

Hair

Epidermis

Sebaceous Gland

Dermis

Subcutis

Venule

Fat Tissue

SKIN

Squamous Cells

Basal Cells

Melanocyte

Sweat Gland

Blood Vessel

Hair Follicle

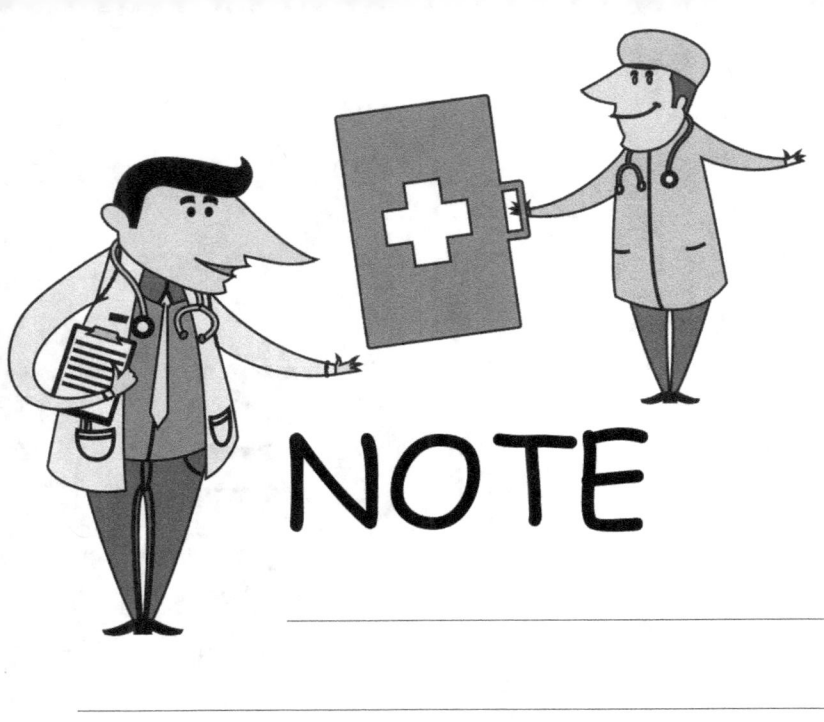

NOTE

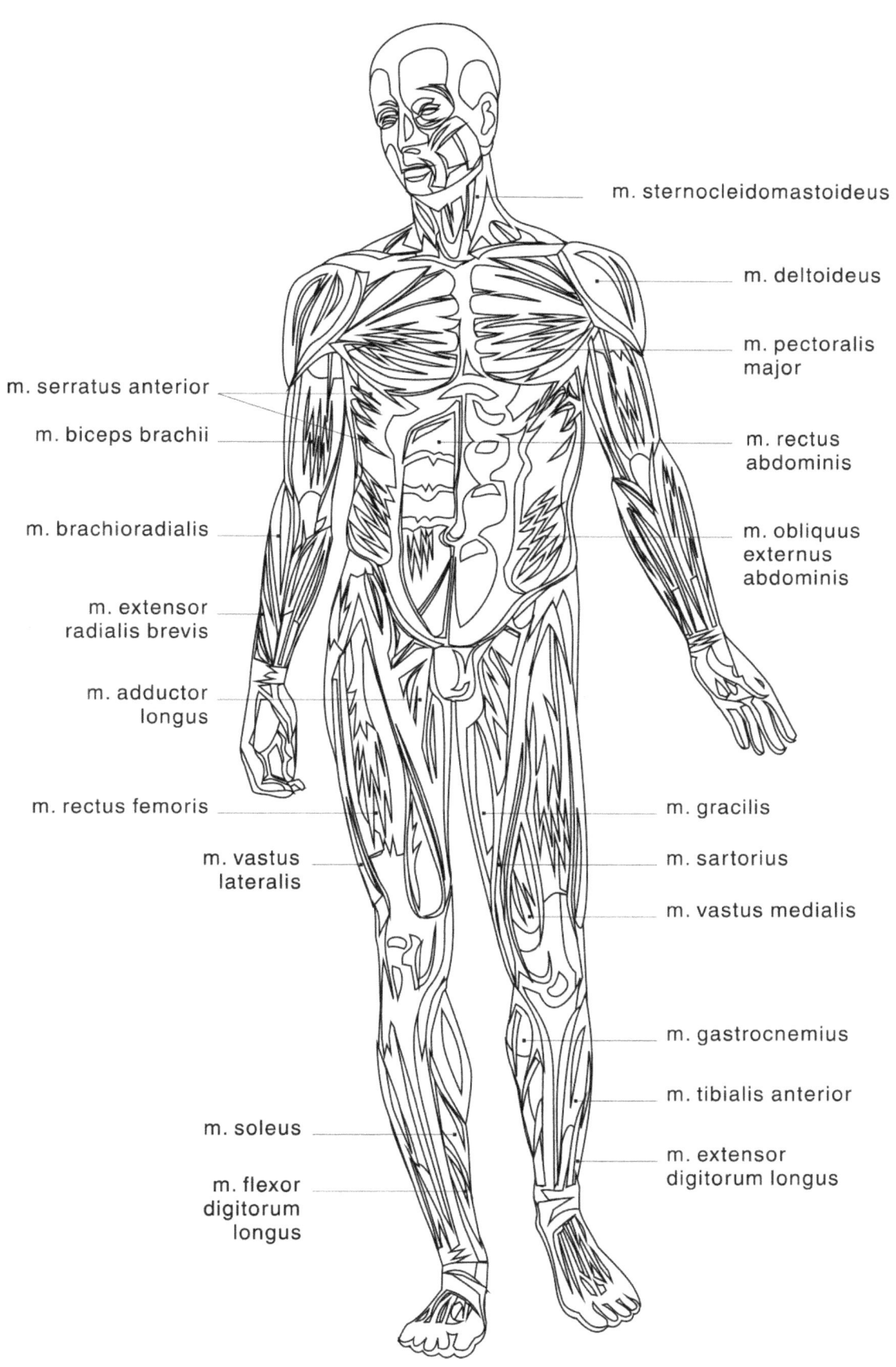

m. sternocleidomastoideus

m. deltoideus

m. pectoralis major

m. serratus anterior

m. biceps brachii

m. rectus abdominis

m. brachioradialis

m. obliquus externus abdominis

m. extensor radialis brevis

m. adductor longus

m. rectus femoris

m. gracilis

m. vastus lateralis

m. sartorius

m. vastus medialis

m. gastrocnemius

m. tibialis anterior

m. soleus

m. extensor digitorum longus

m. flexor digitorum longus

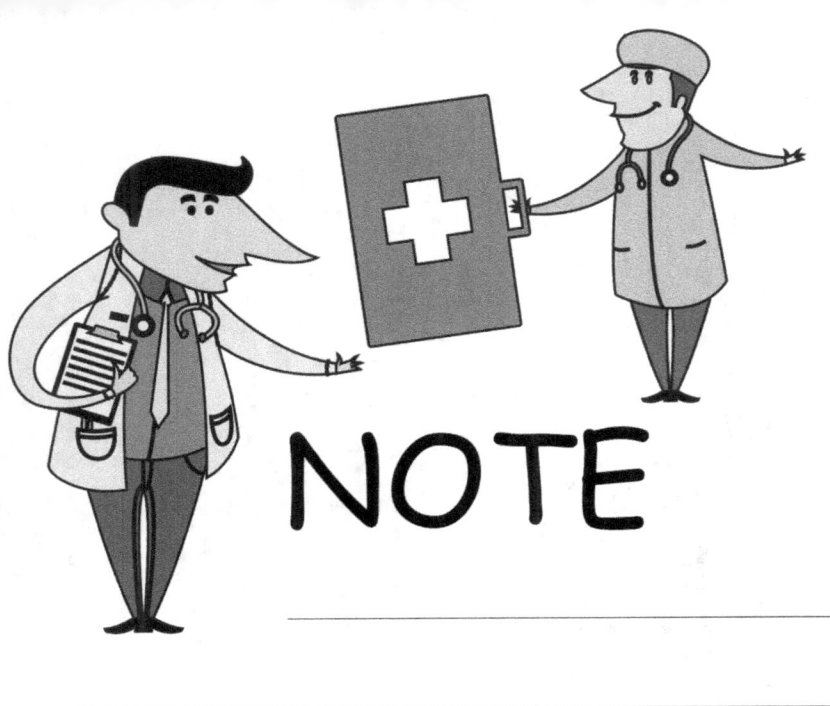

NOTE

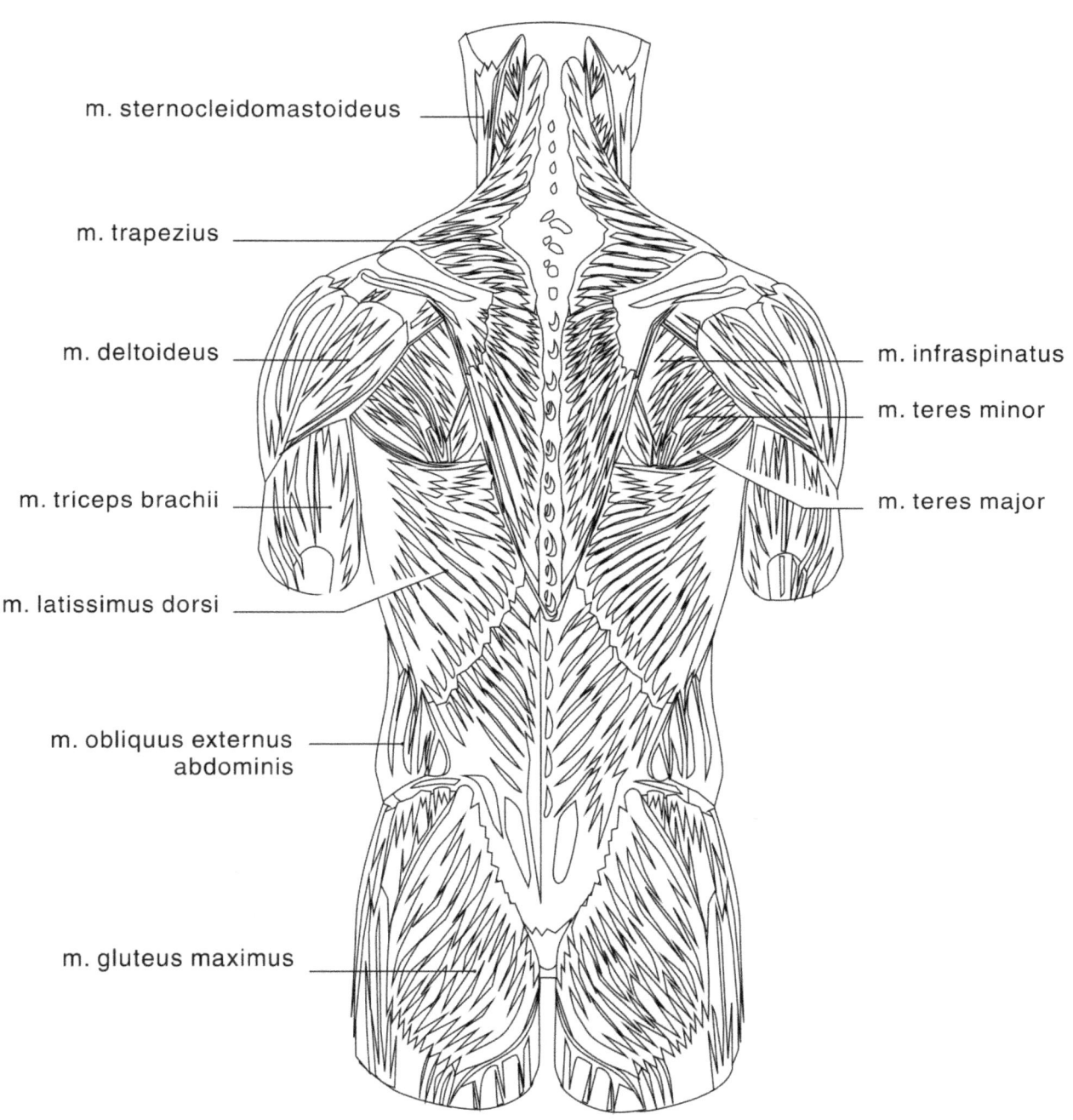

m. sternocleidomastoideus

m. trapezius

m. deltoideus

m. triceps brachii

m. latissimus dorsi

m. obliquus externus
abdominis

m. gluteus maximus

m. infraspinatus

m. teres minor

m. teres major

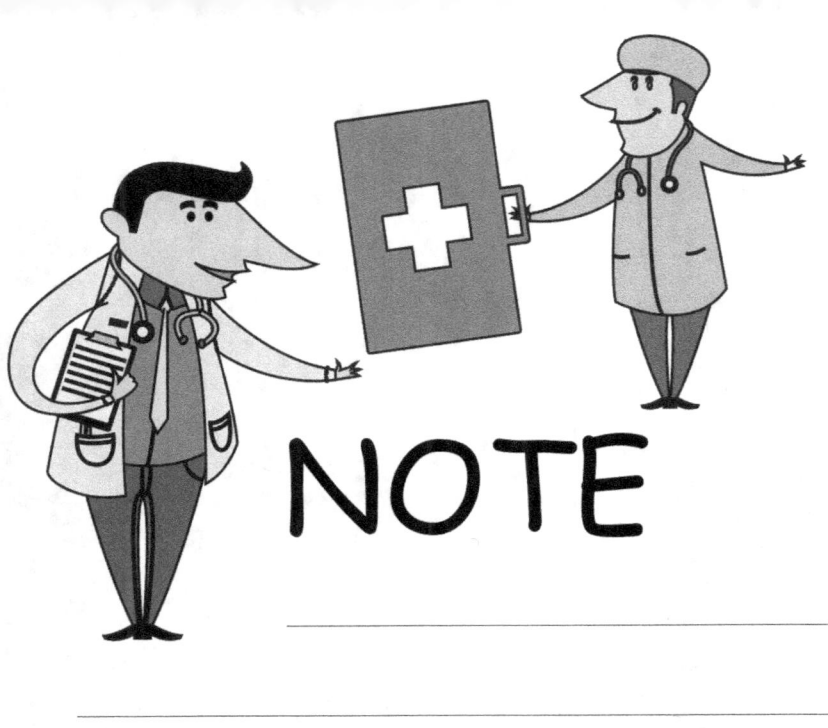

NOTE

ORGANS

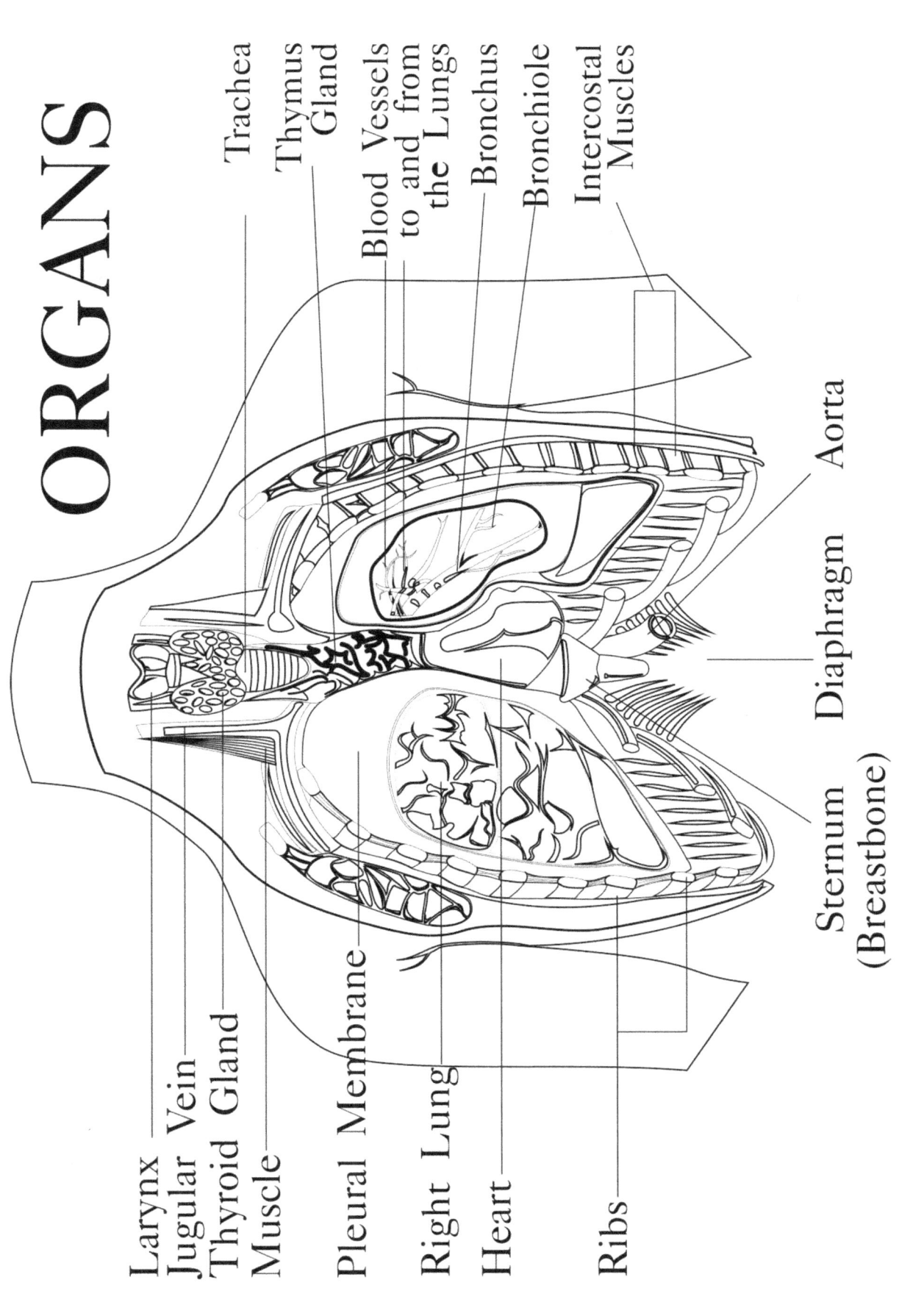

Larynx
Jugular Vein
Thyroid Gland
Muscle

Pleural Membrane

Right Lung

Heart

Ribs

Trachea

Thymus
Gland

Blood Vessels
to and from
the Lungs

Bronchus

Bronchiole

Intercostal
Muscles

Sternum   Diaphragm   Aorta
(Breastbone)

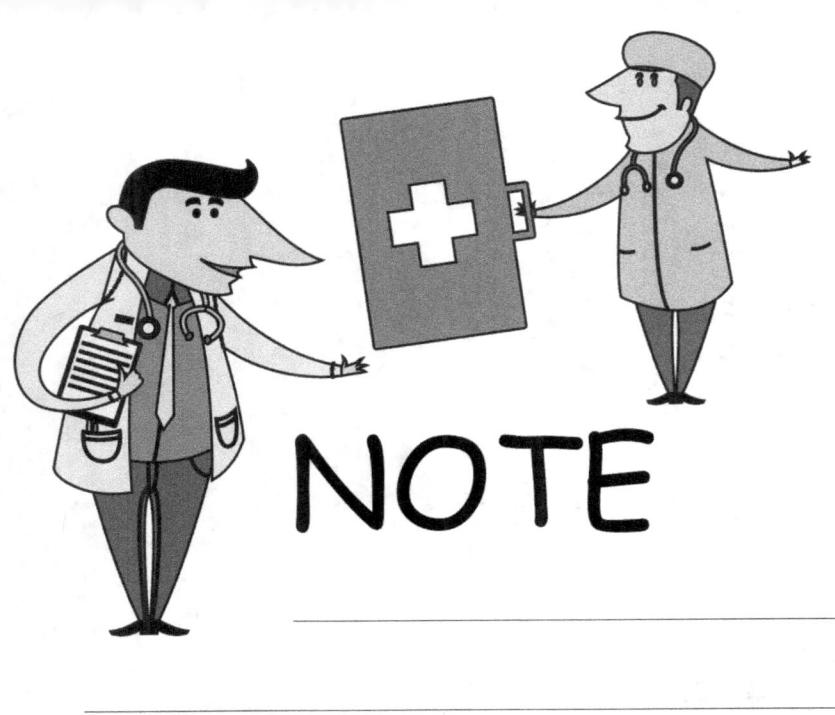

NOTE

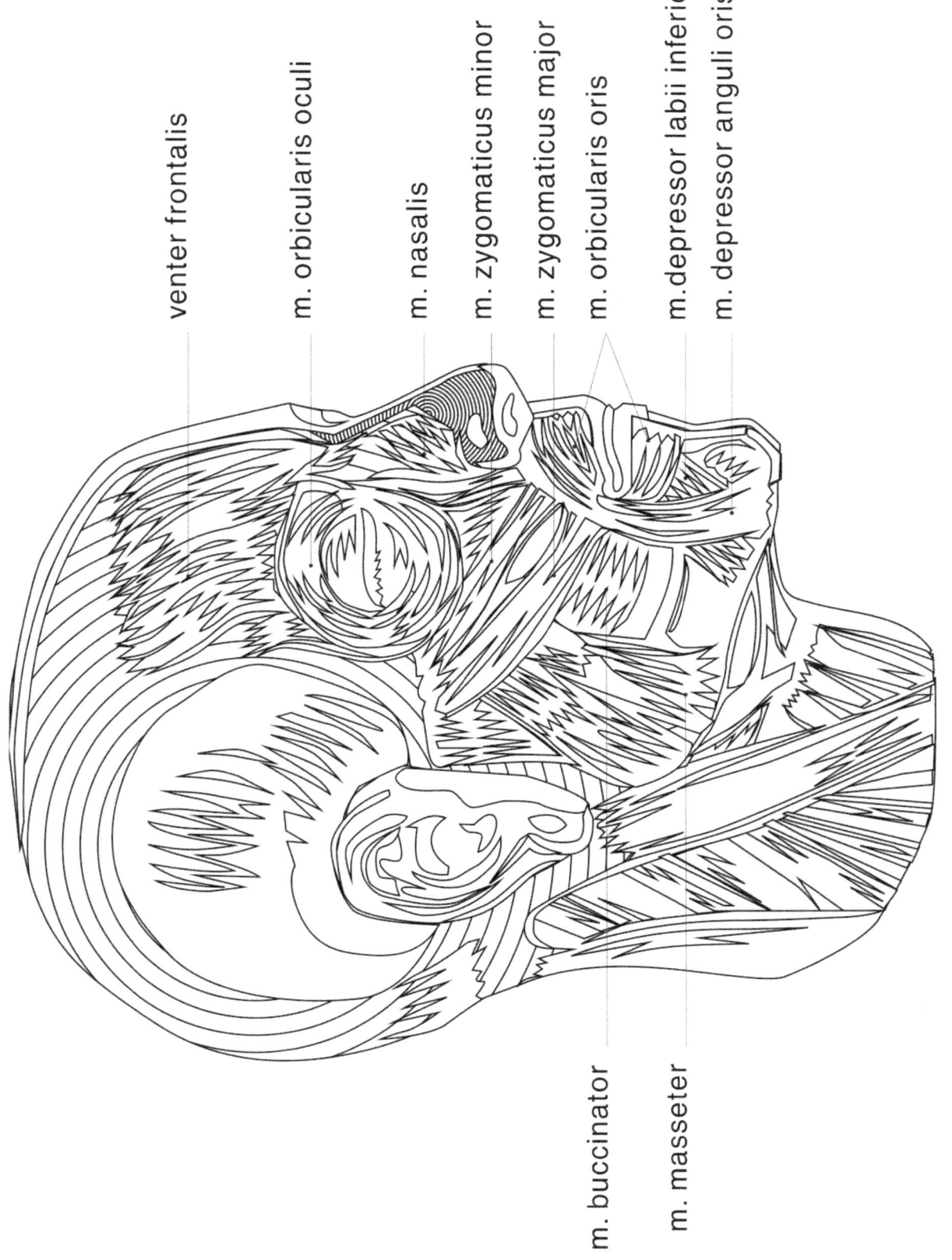

venter frontalis

m. orbicularis oculi

m. nasalis

m. zygomaticus minor

m. zygomaticus major

m. orbicularis oris

m.depressor labii inferioris

m. depressor anguli oris

m. buccinator

m. masseter